SHIATSU THERAPY

The Complete Book of
SHIATSU THERAPY

Toru Namikoshi

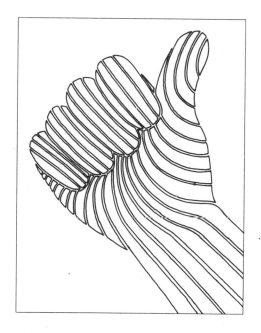

Japan Publications, Inc.

Published by JAPAN PUBLICATIONS, INC., Tokyo

Distributors:
UNITED STATES: *Kodansha International/USA, Ltd., through Harper & Row, Pub-
lishers, Inc., 10 East 53rd Street, New York, 10022.* SOUTH AMERICA:
Harper & Row, Publishers, Inc., International Department. CANADA: *Fitzhenry &
Whiteside Ltd., 150 Lesmill Road, Don Mills, Ontario M3B 2T6.* MEXICO AND
CENTRAL AMERICA: *HARLA S.A. de C. V., Apartado 30–546, Mexico 4, D. F.*
BRITISH ISLES: *International Book Distributors Ltd., 66 Wood Lane End, Hemel
Hempstead, Herts HPZ 4RG.* EUROPEAN CONTINENT: *Boxer books, Inc., Limmat-
strasse 111, 8031 Zurich.* AUSTRALIA AND NEW ZEALAND: *Book Wise (Australia)
Pty Ltd., 104–8 Sussex Street, Sydney 2000.* THE FAR EAST AND JAPAN:
Japan Publications Trading Co., Ltd., 1–2–1, Sarugaku-cho, Chiyoda-ku, Tokyo 101.

First edition: February 1981

LCCC No. 79–1963
ISBN 0–87040–461–X

Printed in Japan by Kyodo Printing Co., Ltd.

Preface

Shiatsu strives first of all to prevent illness and, by calling forth innate self-curative powers, to develop bodies capable of resisting sickness. Even today, when startling technological progress is stripping the veils of mystical secrecy from our universe, many areas of the human body remain only vaguely understood by the most sophisticated medical specialists. As one noted Western doctor has said, all medical textbooks are things of the past. The suffering body of the patient in front us is the medical text of tomorrow. To this statement, which ought to be born in mind always by all people engaged in therapeutical work, I should like to add a thought about the unique nature of each patient.

Though illnesses may be named and the most exhaustive and careful data entered on medical records, the individual patient and his illness cannot be categorized in the kind of broad, clear-cut generalities that dominate modern medicine. The foundation of shiatsu treatment is the belief that each individual case must be regarded as unique. By adjusting treatment to subtle variations in the individual's condition, it is possible to stimulate the body's miraculous self-healing powers and to cultivate both mental and physical well-being.

This book sets forth all of the techniques of practical shiatsu treatment. In addition, however, it provides the reader with the basic knowledge of the structure and functioning of the human body that is a prerequisite to effective shiatsu. It outlines the locations, junctions, and movement points of muscles and nerves. It further shows the paths through which blood vessels and nerves pass, the locations and functions of the organs of the endocrine system, the surface reflex zones and their relations to internal organs, and the causes and natures of pathological states. Overall understanding of these physiological aspects of health and sickness is the basis of a firm grasp of the functional connection between the basic shiatsu-pressure points located in all parts of the body and physiology. This knowledge, in turn, clarifies the effects of shiatsu therapy.

To ensure that this book makes both the basics and the practice of shiatsu as lucid as possible, I have taken the greatest care in selecting a vast amount of photographic illustrative material and in preparing myself charts and drawings to give the reader a clear picture of the relation between shiatsu therapy points and the organization of the body. I believe that, in the richness of its illustrations and the thoroughness and scope of its presentation, this book is revolutionary in the field of shiatsu literature. It is my hope that, through it, I can help more people understand shiatsu therapy accurately, master its techniques, and in this way promote better daily health in themselves and in others.

November 1980   TORU NAMIKOSHI

Contents

Chapter 4:   Therapy for a Kneeling Patient

Chapter 6: Treating Specific Pathological Conditions

Basic Shiatsu Points (anterior)

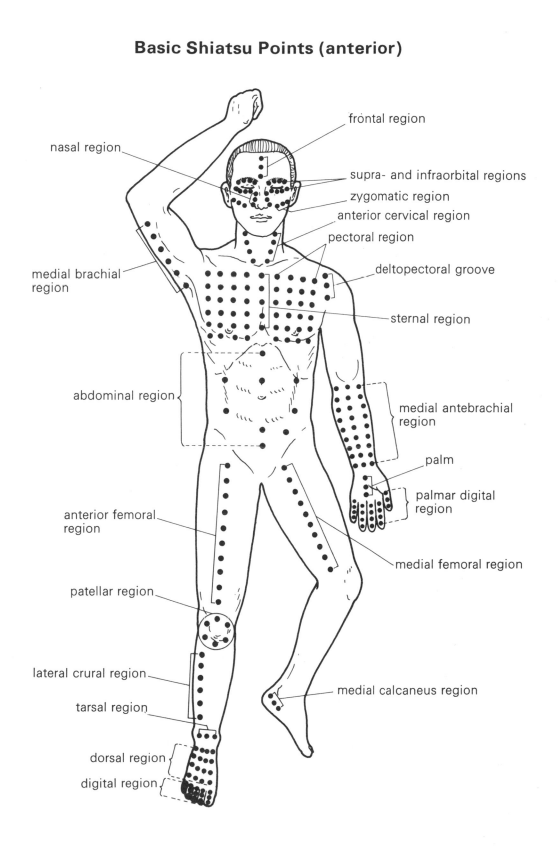

nasal region

frontal region

supra- and infraorbital regions

zygomatic region

anterior cervical region

pectoral region

deltopectoral groove

medial brachial region

sternal region

abdominal region

medial antebrachial region

palm

palmar digital region

anterior femoral region

medial femoral region

patellar region

lateral crural region

tarsal region

medial calcaneus region

dorsal region

digital region

Basic Shiatsu Points (posterior)

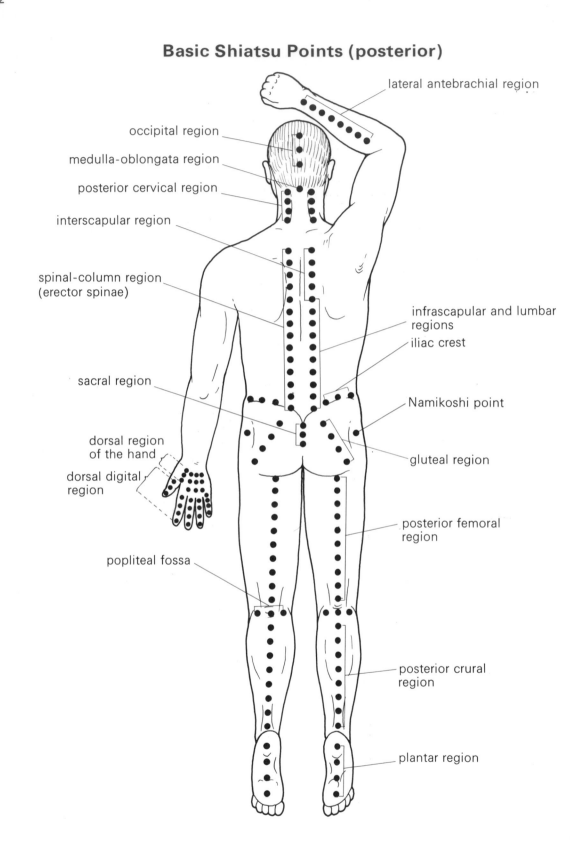

lateral antebrachial region

occipital region

medulla-oblongata region

posterior cervical region

interscapular region

spinal-column region
(erector spinae)

sacral region

dorsal region
of the hand

dorsal digital
region

popliteal fossa

infrascapular and lumbar
regions

iliac crest

Namikoshi point

gluteal region

posterior femoral
region

posterior crural
region

plantar region

Basic Shiatsu Points (lateral)

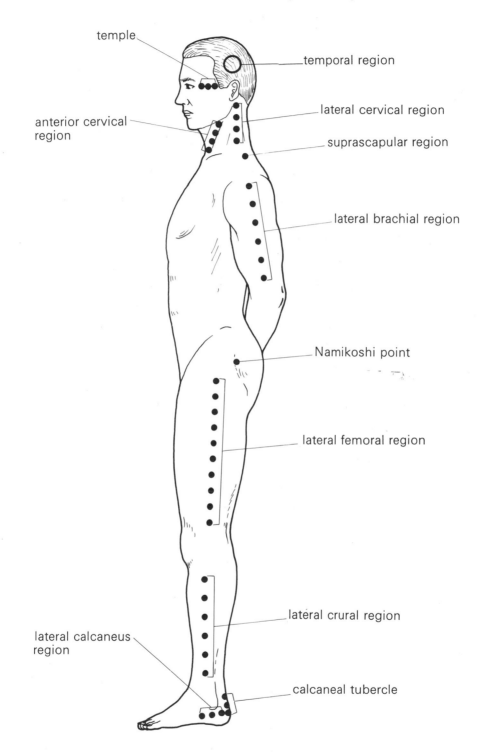

temple

temporal region

anterior cervical region

lateral cervical region

suprascapular region

lateral brachial region

Namikoshi point

lateral femoral region

lateral crural region

lateral calcaneus region

calcaneal tubercle

Muscle and Nerve Points for Motor Reflex to Electric Stimuli

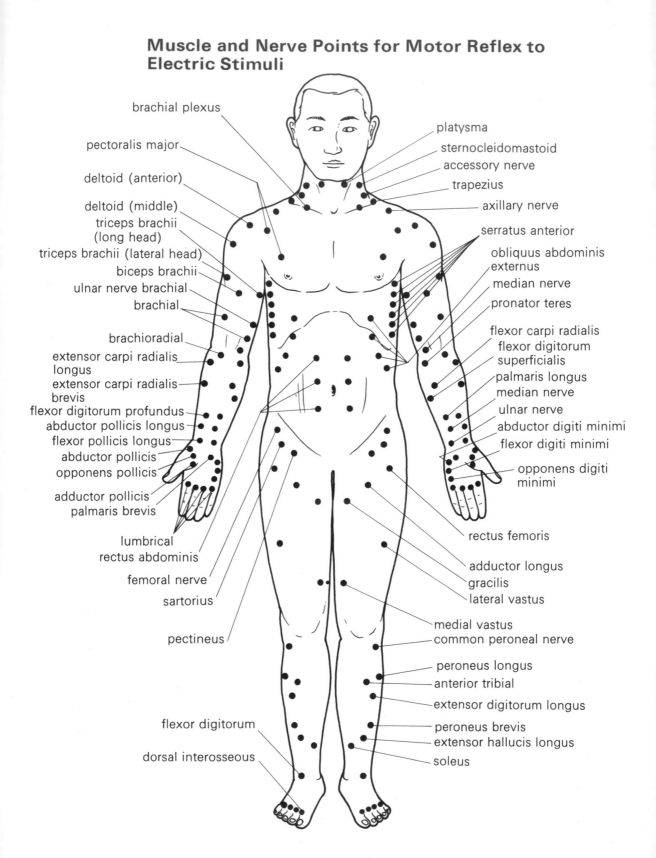

brachial plexus

platysma

pectoralis major

sternocleidomastoid

accessory nerve

deltoid (anterior)

trapezius

deltoid (middle)

axillary nerve

triceps brachii (long head)

serratus anterior

triceps brachii (lateral head)

obliquus abdominis externus

biceps brachii

median nerve

ulnar nerve brachial

pronator teres

brachial

flexor carpi radialis

brachioradial

flexor digitorum superficialis

extensor carpi radialis longus

palmaris longus

extensor carpi radialis brevis

median nerve

flexor digitorum profundus

ulnar nerve

abductor pollicis longus

abductor digiti minimi

flexor pollicis longus

flexor digiti minimi

abductor pollicis

opponens pollicis

opponens digiti minimi

adductor pollicis

palmaris brevis

rectus femoris

lumbrical

adductor longus

rectus abdominis

gracilis

femoral nerve

lateral vastus

sartorius

medial vastus

common peroneal nerve

pectineus

peroneus longus

anterior tribial

extensor digitorum longus

flexor digitorum

peroneus brevis

extensor hallucis longus

dorsal interosseous

soleus

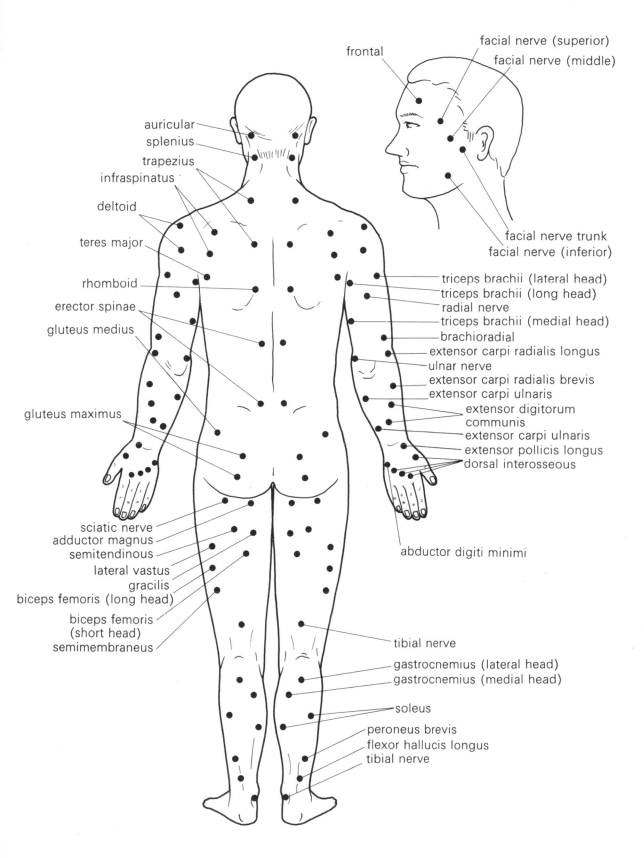

frontal

facial nerve (superior)

facial nerve (middle)

auricular

splenius

trapezius

infraspinatus

deltoid

teres major

rhomboid

erector spinae

gluteus medius

gluteus maximus

facial nerve trunk
facial nerve (inferior)

triceps brachii (lateral head)
triceps brachii (long head)
radial nerve
triceps brachii (medial head)
brachioradial
extensor carpi radialis longus
ulnar nerve
extensor carpi radialis brevis
extensor carpi ulnaris
extensor digitorum
communis
extensor carpi ulnaris
extensor pollicis longus
dorsal interosseous

abductor digiti minimi

sciatic nerve
adductor magnus
semitendinous
lateral vastus
gracilis
biceps femoris (long head)

biceps femoris
(short head)
semimembraneus

tibial nerve

gastrocnemius (lateral head)
gastrocnemius (medial head)

soleus

peroneus brevis
flexor hallucis longus
tibial nerve

Musculature (anterior)

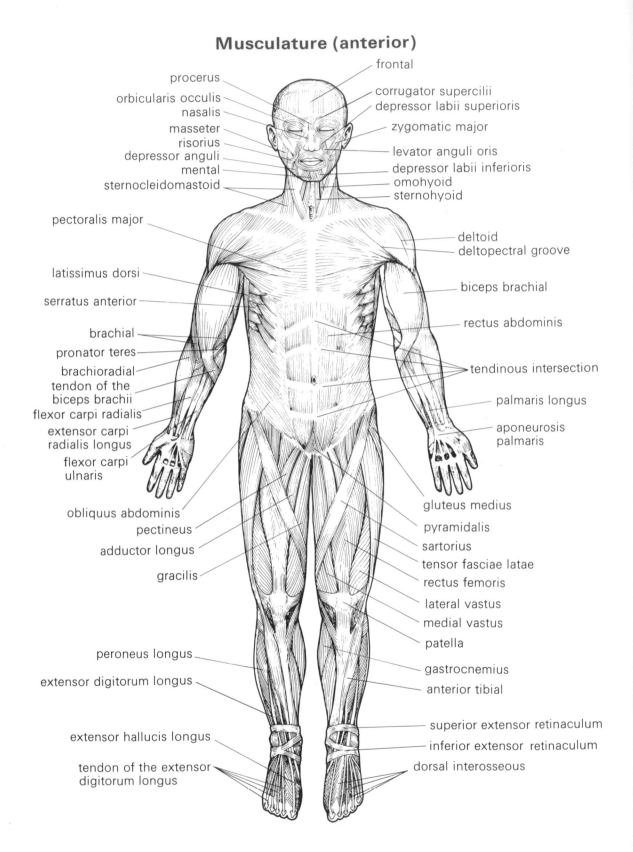

procerus

orbicularis occulis

nasalis

masseter

risorius

depressor anguli

mental

sternocleidomastoid

pectoralis major

latissimus dorsi

serratus anterior

brachial

pronator teres

brachioradial

tendon of the biceps brachii

flexor carpi radialis

extensor carpi radialis longus

flexor carpi ulnaris

obliquus abdominis

pectineus

adductor longus

gracilis

peroneus longus

extensor digitorum longus

extensor hallucis longus

tendon of the extensor digitorum longus

frontal

corrugator supercilii

depressor labii superioris

zygomatic major

levator anguli oris

depressor labii inferioris

omohyoid

sternohyoid

deltoid

deltopectral groove

biceps brachial

rectus abdominis

tendinous intersection

palmaris longus

aponeurosis palmaris

gluteus medius

pyramidalis

sartorius

tensor fasciae latae

rectus femoris

lateral vastus

medial vastus

patella

gastrocnemius

anterior tibial

superior extensor retinaculum

inferior extensor retinaculum

dorsal interosseous

Musculature (posterior)

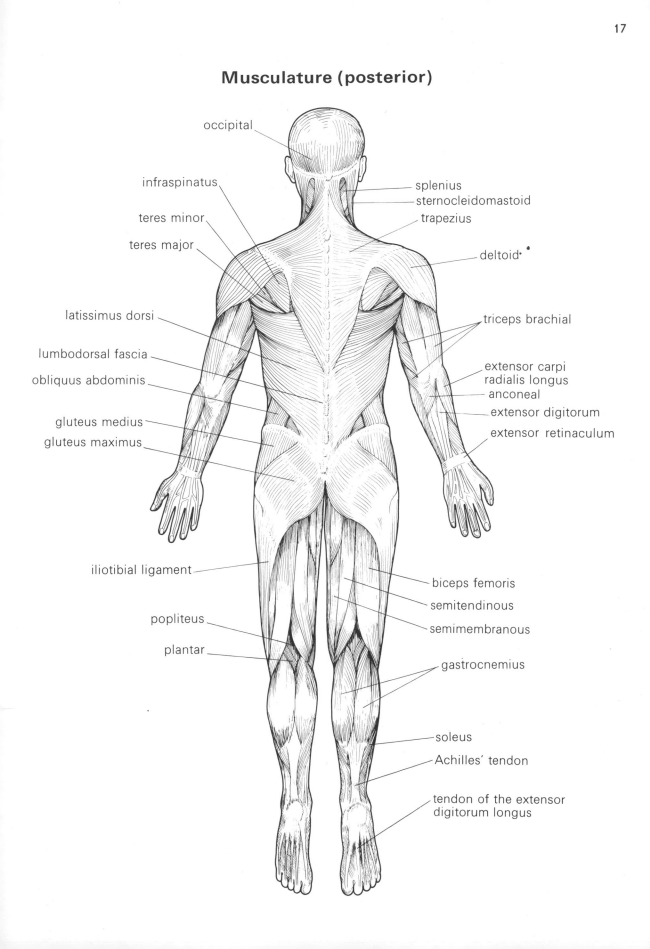

occipital

infraspinatus

teres minor

teres major

latissimus dorsi

lumbodorsal fascia

obliquus abdominis

gluteus medius

gluteus maximus

iliotibial ligament

popliteus

plantar

splenius
sternocleidomastoid
trapezius

deltoid·

triceps brachial

extensor carpi
radialis longus
anconeal
extensor digitorum
extensor retinaculum

biceps femoris
semitendinous
semimembranous

gastrocnemius

soleus
Achilles' tendon

tendon of the extensor
digitorum longus

18

Skeleton

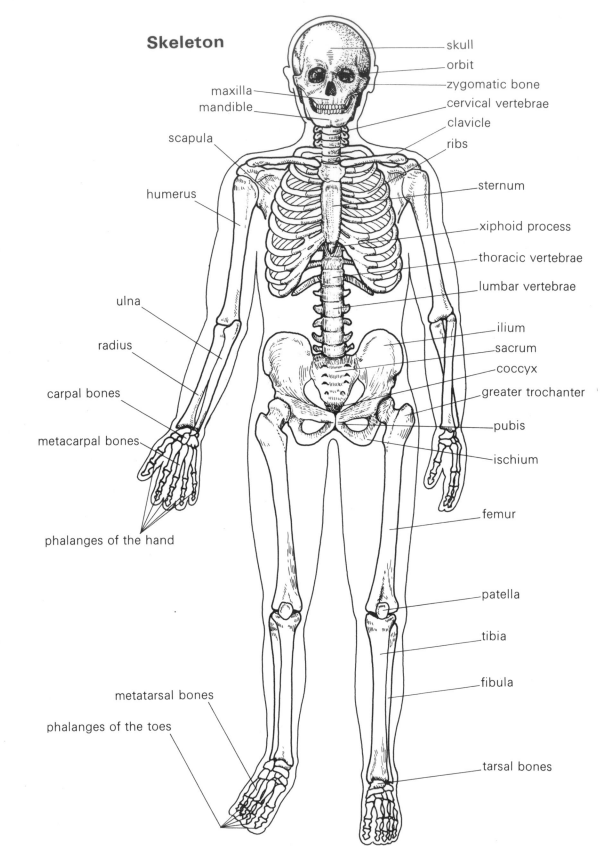

skull
orbit
zygomatic bone
cervical vertebrae
clavicle
ribs
sternum
xiphoid process
thoracic vertebrae
lumbar vertebrae
ilium
sacrum
coccyx
greater trochanter
pubis
ischium
femur
patella
tibia
fibula
tarsal bones

maxilla
mandible
scapula
humerus
ulna
radius
carpal bones
metacarpal bones
phalanges of the hand
metatarsal bones
phalanges of the toes

Chapter 1

General Theory

Development of Shiatsu

Tokujirō Namikoshi, the originator of Namikoshi shiatsu therapy, was born on November 3, 1905, in Kagawa Prefecture, on the island of Shikoku; but, at the age of seven, he, with his entire family—father Eikichi, mother Masa, eldest brother Moichi, second brother Masazo, younger brother Haruo, and elder sister Sadako—moved as settlers from the warm climate of the Seto Inland Sea to the severe setting of the northern Japanese island Hokkaido. The move naturally upset their way of life and entailed a grueling journey, especially since transportation was primitive in those days. On the day after they finally arrived, the mother suddenly began to complain of pain in her knees. At first everyone thought it was only the result of the long, unaccustomed travel and failed to take the ailment seriously; but, as time passed, the pain grew worse and spread to her ankles, wrists, elbows, and shoulders to become what is now called multiple rheumatism of the joints.

There was no doctor in the village where they lived. No medicine was available. None of the children could tolerate merely watching their mother suffer, but all they could do was take turns stroking and pressing the parts of her body that hurt. Perhaps the children's desire to help conveyed itself to her, for gradually their mother began to suffer less. As they continued stroking and massaging her, she frequently said to Tokujirō, "Your hands feel best." This praise encouraged the boy to work harder in treating his mother. Though he was ignorant of physiology or anatomy, his sensitive hands and fingers sensed differences in skin condition, heat, and stiffness; and he adjusted his pressing to these variations. First using a ratio of 80 percent rubbing to 20 percent pressing, he soon found that reversing the percentages was more effective. He concentrated on the places that were stiffest and coolest, and soon his mother's condition took a turn for the better. Since he had been pressing on both sides of the middle region of the spine, unknowingly, he had been stimulating the suprarenal body to secrete cortisone, which cures rheumatism. Ultimately, he brought about a complete cure; and this process of unenlightened experimentation taught him the stubborn powers of self-cure built into the human organism. He had been able to stimulate those powers into activity, and this was the birth of his system of shiatsu.

After surmounting various difficulties in his study of amma massage and Western-style massage, in 1925, Tokujirō Namikoshi opened the Shiatsu Institute of Therapy, on Hokkaido. As time went by, some of the people who came for treatment became his students. In 1933, leaving the school in their charge, he went to Tokyo to open another shiatsu institute but learned at once that, to gain wide recognition for shiatsu, he required the cooperation of others. His devotion to his task finally resulted in the establishment of the Japan Shiatsu Institute, on February 11, 1940. Therapy and lectures at the school gained wide recognition for the distinctive effects of shiatsu treatment. In 1955, for the first time, shiatsu was legally approved, though, unreasonably, only as a part of amma massage. Since its founding, the Japan Shiatsu Institute has trained many graduate specialists and, in 1957, under the new name the Japan Shiatsu School, was officially licensed by the minister of health and welfare. It is the first and only school in the country conducting specialist education in this field. In 1964, shiatsu was at last recognized as distinct and independent from amma and other forms of massage.

At present, people who finish two years' training at the Japan Shiatsu School are qualified to take a national examination. If they pass it, they are licensed as specialists in amma, massage, and shiatsu. Including those who studied in the institution when it still bore its old name, more than twenty thousand specialists have graduated from the Namikoshi school. The publication of the book *Shiatsu* in English has carried the fame of this therapy to many other countries, where it has become so widely known that numerous overseas lecture tours are necessary every year.

Characteristics of Shiatsu Therapy

Shiatsu applies manual and digital pressure to the skin with the aim of preventing and curing illness by stimulating the body's natural powers of recuperation, eliminating fatigue-producing elements, and promoting general good health. The following are its major characteristics.

1. Diagnosis and therapy combined. Each application of shiatsu pressure is diagnosis enabling the therapist to treat according to the body's conditions. The hands and fingers of the trained therapist are sensitive enough to detect abnormalities in the skin or muscles or body heat on contact and thus to pinpoint irregularities and determine at once what basic treatment to employ.
2. Using only the hands and fingers, shiatsu calls on the assistance of no mechanical devices or medicines.
3. No side effects. Since the points to be treated, pressure, and length of application are gauged according to the goal, treatment is accompanied by no unpleasantness and produces no such side effects as later muscular pain.
4. No age limits. Shiatsu can be used on people of all ages ranging from young children to the elderly. In the young, it helps strengthen the body; and in adults and people in middle age, it prevents so-called adult diseases and aging.
5. Shiatsu is a health barometer. Regular shiatsu helps detect bodily irregularities and prevent the accumulation of fatigue and the occurrence of illness.
6. Deepens trust and reliance between the patient and the therapist. The determination of the therapist to cure and the recipient's trust in the therapy combine and interact to increase the effectiveness of treatment.
7. Shiatsu is effective because it treats the whole body. Localized treatment may have temporary effects but cannot bring about basic cures. The only way to do this is first to treat the entire body and then to deal with localities showing pathological symptoms. This, the shiatsu way, it always proves effective.

Shiatsu and Physiological Functions

1. Vitalizing the Skin

Structure of the Skin

The human body is covered with from 1.5 to 2 square meters of skin consisting of an outer layer called the epidermis, a central layer called the corium, and an innermost layer called the subcutaneous tissues. Because of the nerve endings located in it, the skin is able to perceive tactile stimuli, pressure, thermal conditions, and pain. In about one square centimeter of skin there are twenty-five sensory bodies detecting tactile stimuli, from none to three detecting heat, from six to twenty-three detecting cold, and from one hundred to two hundred detecting pain. The other sensations felt by the skin—itchiness, ticklishness, numbness, and so on—are not the results of special perceptors, but compound, mixed, reflex responses to exterior stimuli. Sense receptors in the skin include Meissner's (tactile) corpuscles, Pacinian (lamellated) corpuscles, Krause's corpuscles, Ruffini's corpuscles, and free nerve endings.

Meissner's corpuscles

These receptors for light touch consist of numerous overlapping tactile cells enclosed in a connective tissue capsule and are located in the papillae of the corium. They are plentiful in the palms of the hand, the soles of the feet, and the tips of the fingers.

Fig. 1   Anatomy of the Skin

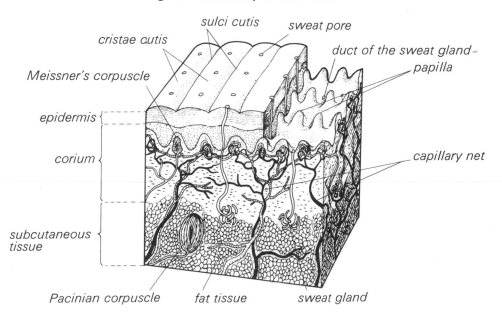

Fig. 2   Sense Receptors

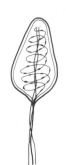

Meissner's corpuscle
—receptor for light tactile

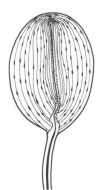

Pacinian corpuscle
—receptor for deep pressure

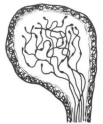

Krause's corpuscle
—receptor for cold

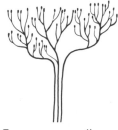

Ruffini's corpuscle
—receptor for heat

Free nerve ending
—receptor for pain

Pacinian corpuscles

These receptors for deep pressure, which consist of layers resembling those of the cross section of an onion, are located in the zone between the corium and the subcutaneous layer and in the subcutaneous layer itself.

Krause's corpuscles

These receptors for cold are located near the upper layer of the corium.

Ruffini's corpuscles

Receptors for heat, Ruffini's corpuscles are located in the corium.

Free nerve endings

These fine endings of numerous nerve branches are pain receptors.

Functions of the Skin

1.   The pigment known as melanin, located in the mucous coat of the epidermis, protects the body from powerful or harmful rays in sunlight, while the resilient corium protects from external percussion.

2.   The skin stores fat and water. The secretions of the sweat and sebaceous

glands nourish the skin and prevent it from drying out. Subcutaneous fat protects from cold and from external percussion.

3. Because of blood circulation and the secretions of the sweat glands, the skin helps control body temperature.

4. The sweat and sebaceous glands remove unwanted substances from the body and contribute to respiration (only about 0.6 percent of the total).

5. Perceptor organs in the skin warn against danger from without.

6. Solar ultraviolet rays are absorbed through the skin to produce vitamin D and thus prevent rickets.

Skin Color

The corneum of the outer epiderms produces new skin cells, and the old dead ones are discarded, some in the form of dandruff and some in flakes that are a cause of the ring around the bathtub left after a person has bathed. Melanin in the mucous coat of the epidermis determines skin color: the greater the amount of melanin, the darker the skin.

Skin Thickness

The thickness of the epidermis varies slightly from part to part. On an average it is from 0.1 to 0.3 millimeters thick. On the eyelids, forehead, and neck, it is from 0.04 to 0.1 millimeters; on the palms, from 0.6 to 1.2 millimeters; on the soles, from 1.7 to 2.8 millimeters. It is thickest on the heels.

The corium, which averages from 1.7 to 2.8 millimeters is only 0.6 millimeters on the eyelids, 1.5 millimeters on the forehead, and 2 millimeters on the head. It is from 4 to 5 millimeters thick on the neck.

Subcutaneous fat is the thickest part of the skin, where it is present at all. It is best developed on the buttocks, the abdomen, the cheeks, and the female breasts. Fat tissues are absent on the eyelids and on the scrotum and penis of the male and the labia minora of the female.

Shiatsu Effects on Sweat and Sebaceous Glands

Sweat glands on the human body are of two kinds: the eccrine glands, which are distributed all over the body; and the apocrine glands, which are numerous in the armpits and the vicinity of the genitalia and which produce a stronger-smelling secretion than the eccrine glands.

The sebaceous glands, located above the hair roots, secrete an oily substance called sebum. They are not found in such hairless zones as the palms and soles. The pimples of puberty are caused by oversecretion of sebum and consequent clogging of the hair pouches, which become infected. Once the infection is cured, the skin recovers its natural softeness and resilience. In old age, subcutaneous fat contracts; and sebaceous glands produce less sebum, with the result that the skin wrinkles and sags. By applying shiatsu directly to the skin it is possible to help prevent this sign of aging.

2.   Limbering the Muscles

Kinds of Muscles

Three kinds of muscles account for an average of about 45 percent of human body weight.

1. *Striated muscles.* Connecting the members of the skeletal system, these muscles are important in movement and maintenance of posture. Since they can be operated deliberately they are sometimes called volunatary muscles. They consist of bundles of fibers arranged in striated patterns. Generally, tonus maintained in these muscles helps the body stay in the desired position. During sleep, however, this tonus is lost, as indicated by the way the head of a seated drowsy person lolls from side to side. There are four hundred striated muscles in the body.

2. *Smooth muscles.* These involunatry muscles contract and expand automatically without volitional control. Forming the walls of the blood vessels and the internal organs, they have short fibers and are unstriated.

3. *The heart muscle.* This involuntary, striated muscles is extremely strong.

Muscular Fatigue

Continued tension or operation of muscles gradually causes accumulation of fatigue-producing elements (lactic acid and carbon dioxide gas) and a resulting induration of the muscle fibers, which lose power to contract. The flow of blood and lymph is thus reduced, and capillary nourishment becomes insufficient. If induration continues, contracture develops. And, if this conditions is not corrected, nerves are dulled; and the internal organs and endocrine system are affected with a consequent loss of bodily balance. As this suggests, the condition usually referred to as stiff muscles can become serious and should be corrected with shiatsu therapy.

Manual Muscle Testing

100%	5	Normal	Complete range of motion against gravity with full resistance.
75%	4	Good	Complete range of motion against gravity with some resistance.
50%	3	Fair	Complete range of motion against gravity.
25%	2	Poor	Complete range of motion with gravity eliminated.
10%	1	Trace	Evidence of slight contractility. No motion.
0%	0	Zero	No evidence of contractility.

3. Stimulating the Circulation of Body Fluids

Since they supply nourishment to and remove wastes from all of the cellular tissues, body fluids—blood, tissue fluid, and lymph—and their good circulation are essential to the life of the cells. Bright red arterial blood is transported from the heart outward to the other parts of the body by means of the aorta, then by means of the auxiliary arteries to the arterioles and ultimately to the millions of capillaries that supply nourishment and oxygen to the cells. Blood then removes wastes from the cells and returns through the venulae and major veins toward the heart in dark red venous form. Before returning to the heart, it passes through the lungs, where it is cleansed and where it receives the supply of oxygen that makes it bright red again. The course outward from the heart to the body cells through the arteries and capillaries is called greater (systemic) circulation. The course back to the heart by way of the lungs and the pulmonary vessels is called lesser (pulmonary) circulation.

Arteries, veins, and lymph vessels do more than transport body fluids. The smooth muscles of their walls contract automatically and control the pressure, speed, distribution, flow, and quantity of the liquid passing through them. In this way, they regulate the load on the heart. When they fail to function as they

Fig. 3   Diagram of the Circulatory System

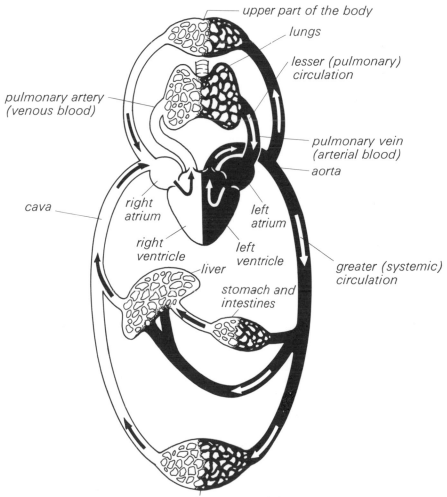

should, circulation of body fluids becomes sluggish, the cells do not receive adequate nourishment, and harmful wastes accumulate. In the case of blood vessels, this strains the heart. Insufficient functioning of the walls of the lymph vessels causes edema.

The posture and state of activity of the body influence circulation. Long standing in one position makes circulation sluggish and causes swelling in the legs. Ordinary walking stimulates muscular contraction, which accelerates the return of blood to the heart through the veins. By activating the operation of the whole body—especially of the carotid sinus—shiatsu stimulates efficient circulation of body fluids. Its pressure operation has good effects on the arms and legs and vitalizes return of venous blood to the heart.

4.   Regulating Neural Functions

The nervous system, which acts like a communications network connecting all parts of the body, is divided into the central nervous system, consisting of the brain, enclosed in the protective casing of the skull, and the spinal cord, enclosed in the vertebral column, and the peripheral nervous system (see Figs. 4 and 5). The peripheral nervous system is made up of the cerebrospinal system (brain and spinal cord) and the autonomic nervous system. The cerebrospinal nervous system—or the mixed nervous system—controls the motor nerves, which move the skeletal muscles, and the sensory nerves, which enable the body to experience pain, heat, cold, and so on. The autonomic system controls those functions and organs over which volition has no sway—circulation, the endocrine system, and the operation of the internal organs—and is made up of the sympathetic and parasympathetic subsystems, which operate in harmony and check each other. For instance, the sympathetic system restrains the operation of the alimentary system, whereas the parasympathetic system stimulates it. When the body is healthy, these two systems act together harmoniously. An abnormality—prolonged nervous stress, for instance—stimulates the brain to emit impulses that travel from the central to the peripheral nervous system and upset the balance of the autonomic system. When this happens, circulation to the vessels of the interior organs is obstructed; and such things as excess secretion of stomach acid resulting in nervous stomachache or even ulcers can take place. Shiatsu treatment on the anterior cervical region, the medulla oblongata, and both sides of the spinal column is important in regulating the autonomic nervous system. The head and the medulla oblongata are vital to regularity in the hypothalamus, the pituitary gland, the pyramidal tract and extrapyramidal system, the cerebral cortex, and other elements of the central nervous system. Since the pyramidal tract and extrapyramidal system help control posture and motion, disorder in them caused by abnormal muscular tension makes such control impossible and can lead to inability to walk and to Parkinson's disease. When cerebral hemorrhage damages the cerebral hemisphere or the pyramidal tract, the opposite side of the body is paralyzed. Such disorders in the nervous system are very hard to cure.

Pathological Signs
Obstruction in the pyramidal tract causes the following abnormal reflex reactions, which are positive.

Functioning of the Autonomic Nervous System

	Tension in the sympathetic nerves	Tension in the para-sympathetic nerves (vagus nerve)
pupil	dilation (opening)	contraction (closing)
eyeball	protrusion	retraction
lacrimal grands	repression of secretion	stimulation of secretion
salivary glands	condensation (reduction in quantity)	dilution (increase in quantity)
heart	stimulation (acceleration)	suppression (deceleration)
blood vessels	contraction	enlargement
coronary artery	enlargement	contraction
blood pressure	increase	lowering
bronchi and trachea	relaxation	contraction (coughing)
stomach—action	supression	acceleration
—secretion	reduction	increase
small and large intestines	suppression of action (suppression of peristalsis)	acceleration of action (speeding of peristalsis)
pancreas	reduction of secretion	increase
gallbladder	relaxation	contraction
medulla of the suprarenal body	acceleration of secretion	
bladder	enlargement (suppression of urination)	contraction (stimulation of urination)
uterus	contraction	relaxation
sweat glands	stimulation of secretion	secretion of light sweat
erector pili muscle	contraction	

Fig. 5 Peripheral Nervous System

Fig. 4 Central Nervous System

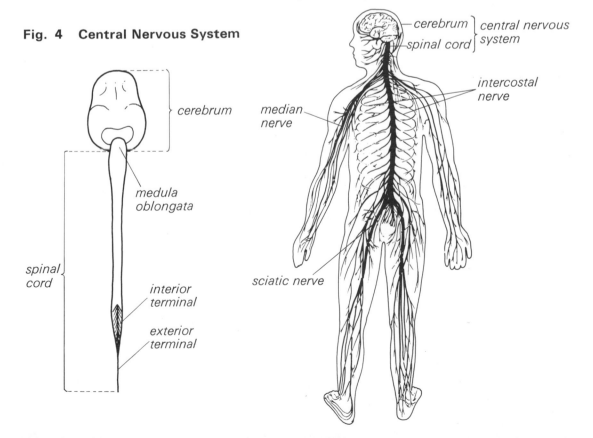

Fig. 6 Pathological Signs

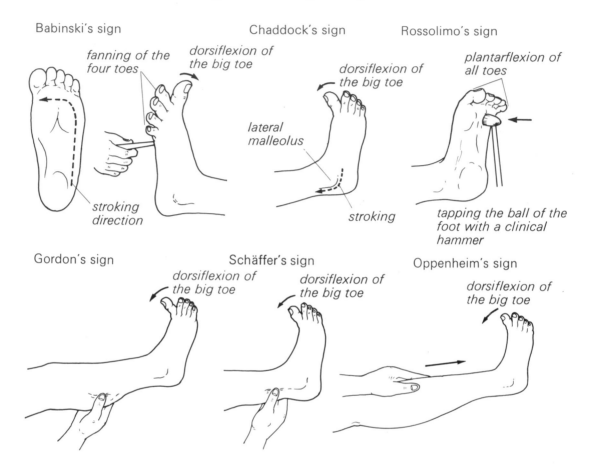

1. *Babinski's sign.* Stroking the outer edge of the sole of the foot with something like the handle of a clinical hammer from the heel toward the toes and across the ball of the foot causes dorsiflexion of the big toe and fanning of the other four toes.

2. *Chaddock's sign.* Stroking the outer edge of the sole with something like the handle of a clinical hammer toward the lateral malleolus causes dorsiflexion of the big toe.

3. *Rossolimo's sign.* Tapping the ball of the foot near the big toe with a clinical hammer causes plantarflexion of all toes.

4. *Gordon's sign.* Firmly squeezing the calf causes dorsiflexion of the big toe.

5. *Schäffer's sign.* Firmly squeezing the Achilles' tendon causes dorsiflexion of the big toe.

6. *Oppenheim's sign.* Strongly stroking downward from the knee along the shin causes dorsiflexion of the big toe.

Reflexes in the Autonomic Nervous System

1. *Carotid-sinus reflexes.* Because of their importance to shiatsu treatment on the anterior cervical region the physiological operations of the carotid sinus area must be thoroughly understood. The carotid sinus is located at the point in the neck where the carotid artery branches, leading to the head. At this point is situated the carotid body, a distribution of nerve tissues connected with the vagus nerve called the sinus nerve. It is extremely sensitive to blood-pressure and respiratory conditions. For instance, when blood pressure becomes high, it reacts by causing the walls of the blood vessels to expand, with the result that reflex dilation lowers the blood pressure and causes brachycardia. Shiatsu point 1 on the anterior cervical region (for points and their locations, refer to chapter three) is located in the carotid sinus. Treatment on this point effectively influences lowering of blood pressure and brachycardia. But pressure must not be prolonged on either of the points and must never be applied to both simultaneously. These points are used in Hering's test to determine symptoms of tension in the vagus nerve. Pulse of more than ten per minute is considered positive.

2. *Aschner's phenomenon.* This reflex is especially important in connection with shiatsu pressure applied to the eyes with the palms. Persistent, gentle pressure applied to the eyes stimulates the endings of the trigeminal nerve located behind them. This in turn stimulates reflexes in the central body of the vagus nerve, thereby reducing pulse and lowering blood pressure. This reflex is employed in Aschner's test. A decrease of more than from ten to fifteen per minute in the pulse rate is considered positive, indicating accelerated tension in the vagus nerve. In shiatsu therapy, gentle—never strong—pressure with the palms is applied to the eyes for no more than ten seconds.

Shiatsu and Cutaneovisceral Reflexes

When irregularities occur in the internal organs, excitation of the afferent visceral sensory nerves operates on the posterior horns of the spinal column, on the autonomic nerves associated with it, or on the sensory nerves of the skin and musculature and thus cause hyperesthesia (Head's zone) and excess muscular tension producing stiffness or pain. This process, called referred pain, is of the upmost importance in diagnosing disorders of the internal organs. How referred pain—which affects the shoulders, legs, back, abdomen, and chest—takes place is not fully understood; but it is possible that nerve fibers transmit organic irregularities directly to the surface of the body in reflexes that do not involve synapse. If this is true, it may be that acetylcholine or some similar transmission substance is secreted in the spinal segments of the posterior horns that ought to connect by synapse with the visceral sensory nerves and thus stimulates nervous impulse. This impulse in turn excites sensory nerves associated with those spinal segments. In accordance with this concept, shiatsu applied to the oversensitive or muscularly tense parts of the surface of the body should set up the reverse process. In other words, according to its force and duration, pressure applied to the surface of the body should set up reflexes in the internal organs, stimulating them to function as they should and thus curing irregularities.

Fig. 7 Locations for Shiatsu Application for the Spinal Nervous System and Cutaneovisceral Reflexes

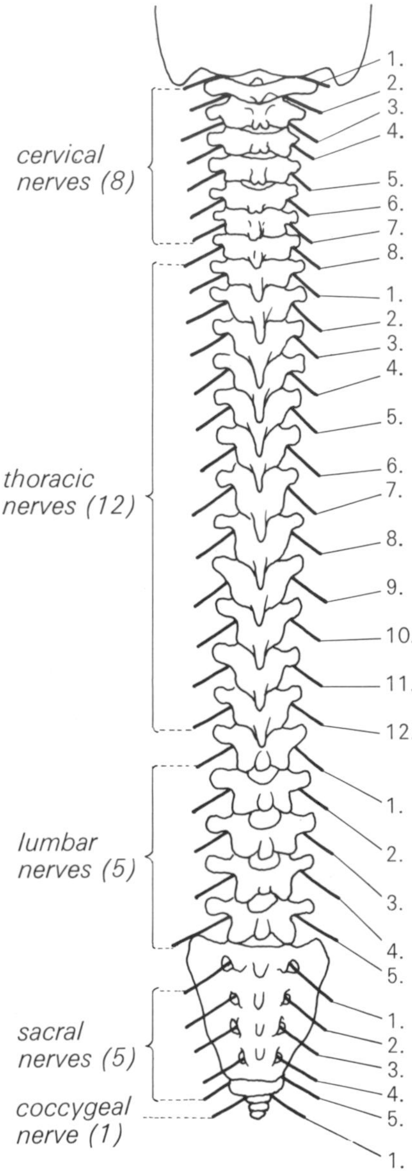

cervical nerves (8)

1. Vertebral artery, eyes, throat, submandibular gland
2. Vertebral artery, larynx, eyes, sublingual gland
3. Heart, lungs, diaphragm, vertebral artery
4. Thyroid gland, diaphragm, vasomotor nerves, vertebral artery, trachea, esophagus
5. Thyroid gland, heart, diaphragm, vertebral artery, trachea, esophagus
6. Vertebral artery, trachea, esophagus, heart, lungs
7. Trachea, esophagus, eyes, lungs, heart
8. Eyes, lungs, trachea, bronchi, heart

thoracic nerves (12)

1. Eyes, ears, heart, lungs, pleura, vasomotor nerves, bronchi
2. Vasomotor nerves, intercostal nerves, pleura, heart, bronchi
3. Intercostal nerves, heart, lungs, pleura, liver, diaphragm, bronchi
4. Intercostal nerves, heart, lungs, pleura, diaphragm, trachea, mammary glands
5. Intercostal nerves, mammary glands, pleura, stomach, spleen, diaphragm, liver
6. Pleura, stomach, spleen, intercostal nerves, diaphragm, liver
7. Intercostal nerves, peritoneum, stomach, spleen, gallbladder, liver, pancreas
8. Intercostal nerves, peritoneum, stomach, spleen, bile duct, gallbladder, pancreas, suprarenal glands
9. Intercostal nerves, vasomotor nerves, suprarenal glands, pancreas, small intestine
10. Intercostal nerves, peritoneum, pancreas, spleen, bile duct, diaphragm, urinary tract, kidneys
11. Peritoneum, diaphragm, pancreas, kidneys, urinary tract, large intestine small intestine
12. Peritoneum, diaphragm, kidneys, urinary tract, large intestine, small intestine, appendix

lumbar nerves (5)

1. Small intestine, appendix, uterus, ovaries, Fallopian tubes, testes, penis, bladder
2. Large intestine, small intestine, appendix, uterus, ovaries, testes, penis, ejaculatory duct
3. Uterus, ovaries, Fallopian tubes, prostate gland, ejaculatory duct, testes, penis, bladder
4. Rectum, anus, prostate gland, bladder, uterus, sigmoid colon
5. Bladder, prostate gland, rectum, testes, uterus, sigmoid colon

sacral nerves (5)

1. Bladder, anus, erection, emission, rectum, vagina, cervix of uterus
2. Bladder, anus, erection, emission, rectum, vagina, cervix of uterus
3. Bladder, anus, erection, emission, rectum, vagina, cervix of uterus
4. Bladder, anus, vagina, erection, emission, cervix of uterus
5. Bladder, anus, vagina, erection, emission, cervix of uterus

coccygeal nerve (1)

1. Anal area and coccyx perceptions

Practical experience and operation expedience have established four points in the posterior cervical region, five in the interscapular region, ten from the infrascapular to the lumbar regions, and three in the sacral region for shiatsu therapy. A practitioner will find, however, that, through repeated applications he makes small upward or downward adjustments with the result that all of the thirty-one points listed above are treated. This kind of therapy restores harmony to the autonomic nervous system.

5.   Controlling the Endocrine System

By secreting a variety of different hormones directly into the blood and in this way preserving chemical balance and connection among internal organs, the endocrine system is vital to maintenance of normal health. The name *hormone* for the substances secreted by the ductless glands of the system derives from a Greek word meaning to excite or stimulate. This indicates the nature of the role they play. Reductions or increases of the small amounts of hormones produced retard or stimulate the functioning of internal organs.

Fig. 8   Endocrine Glands

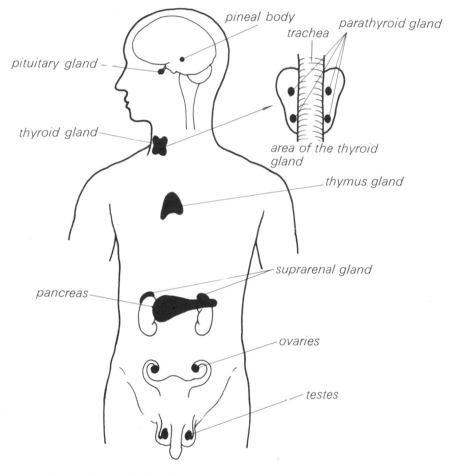

Functions of the Glands

1.   *Pituitary gland.* Each of the three lobes—anterior, median, and posterior—of the pituitary gland secretes a number of hormones.

Anterior lobe: the growth hormone (GH); the adrenocorticotrophic hormone (ACTH); the thyroid-stimulating hormone (TSH); the gonadotrophic hormone including the luteinizing hormone (LH), which stimulates the production of sperm cells in the male and ova in the females, and the follicle-stimulating hormone (FSH).

Median lobe: Melanophorin (MSH), related to the melanin bodies, which are not thoroughly understood.

Posterior lobe: Pituitorin, which operates on the contraction of the blood vessels and the uterus and which suppresses diuresis. Reduction in the secretion of this hormone causes excess urination and can result in diabetes insipidus.

Shiatsu applied to the medulla oblongata point has an effect on the functioning of the pituitary gland. In this case, pressure application is somewhat prolonged.

2. *Thyroid gland.* Thyroxine, secreted by the thyroid gland, which is situated under the front part of the thyroid cartilage, stimulates metabolism. Lack of this hormone slows down metabolism and cause sluggishness, swelling in the face and other parts of the body, and myxedema. Overproduction of thyroxine results in loss of weight, protruding eyeballs, irregularity in heart functioning, and Basedow's disease. The thyroid gland operates in connection with the anterior lobe of the pituitary gland, and shiatsu for it is applied to points 3 and 4 of the anterior cervical region and to the medulla oblongata.

3. *Parathyroid glands.* The parathyroid hormone, secreted from the two parathyroid glands located on each side of the underside of the thyroid gland, helps make use of the calcium in the blood. A low production of this hormone causes insufficient calcium in the body, abnormal excitation of the cells of the nervous system, and tonic spasm of all the body muscles (tetany).

Shiatsu for this gland is applied to points 3 and 4 of the anterior cervical region and to the medulla oblongata.

4. *Suprarenal bodies.* Attached to the upper points of the left and right kidneys, the suprarenal bodies consist of a cortex and a medullary substance. Adrenalin secreted from the medullary substance affects the sympathetic nervous system, stimulates the heart, dilates the muscles of the bronchi, and stimulates contraction of blood vessels. In addition, it helps counter stress. The cortex secretes more than forty hormones of the corticoid system, which, by regulating ACTH secreted by the pituitary gland, provide bodily resistance. Reduction of the secretion of these hormones results in Addison's disease, myasthenia, and rheumatism. Oversecretion of them causes obesity and diabetes. Shiatsu related to the suprarenal bodies is applied to points 3, 4, and 5 in the infrascapular region; prolonged palm pressure and vibrating pressure are employed.

5. *Pancreas.* Through its efferent vessel, the pancreas secretes digestive fluid —which is not a hormone—into the duodenum. But the millions of special cells called islets of Langerhans distributed throughout the pancreas tissues secrete insulin, which lowers blood-sugar levels. Insufficient secretion of insulin results in diabetes. The diaphragm and points 1, 2, and 3 in the infrascapular region are the locations for shiatsu applications in connection with the pancreas.

6. *Sexual glands.* The male hormone (androgen) and the female hormone (estrogen), secreted from among the cells of the ovaries and testes, stimulate male and female characteristics respectively and cause growth and development of the sexual organs after the start of puberty. These glands operate in connection with the pituitary gland. The sacral region, the inguinal region, the lower abdominal region, and the medulla oblongata are the zones for shiatsu.

7. *The pineal body and the thymus.* The small pineal body, located between the cerebrum and the cerebellum, regulates bodily growth and the development of sexual organs but ceases to function once the body has reached full growth.

Situated behind the sternum, the thymus, like the pineal body, is said, to regulate body growth. It disappears as the body develops.

6. Skeletal System

Bones

The two hundred bones in the human body—twenty-six in the spine, twenty-five in the chest, twenty-three in the skull, sixty-four in the arms, and sixty-two in the legs—are connected by tendons and ligaments in fixed arrangements to create the skeletal system. The bones are categorized by forms: long bones, short bones, flat bones, pneumatic bones, and so on. The long bones, found mainly in the arms and legs, including the humerus, radius, ulna, femur, tibia, and fibula, consist of a diaphysis and a bulbous or curved epiphysis (see Fig. 9). Nutrient foramens, through which blood vessels pass, run through the diaphysis. The numbers and directions of these foramens are fixed according to bone type; for instance, they run downward in the femur and upward in the humerus. The short bones lack a clearly defined diaphysis and epiphysis and are irregular in shape: carpal and tarsal bones and the vertebrae are examples. Flat bones include the platelike parietal and occipital bones. Pneumatic bones are hollow and air-filled; the frontal bone and the maxilla are examples.

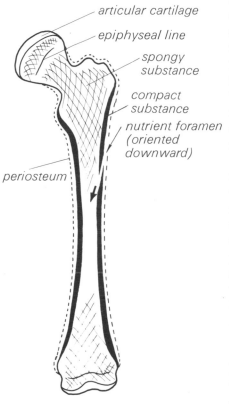

articular cartilage
epiphyseal line
spongy substance
compact substance
nutrient foramen (oriented downward)
periosteum

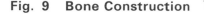

Fig. 9   Bone Construction

Bone Structure

Bones consist of the following parts: periosteum, bony substance (compact and spongy), cartilage, and marrow. The periosteum, a tough double membrane made of connective tissues and rich in blood vessels and nerves, covers and protects the outer surface of the bone, assists in growth and regeneration, and provides nourishment. The compact substance is hard, dense, and solid. The spongy substance is riddled with small lacunae. In general, the exterior of the bone is a thin layer of compact substance covering the spongy substance beneath. But, in long bones, the diaphysis consists of compact substance only; and the epiphysis consists of spongy substance with a compact-substance covering. Haversian canals in the dense, compact substance permit the passage of blood vessels and nerves. The holes in the bony substance in the spongy substance are arranged in an orderly fashion to provide maximum resistance against exterior forces.

Between the diaphysis and the epiphysis of long bones are layers of cartilage permitting growth by cellular reproduction and gradual ossification. The extremities of bones articulating with adjacent bones are cartilage for smooth movement and shock absorption. Marrow fills the marrow cavity in the dia-physis of long bones and small cavities in the spongy substance. Blood cells are produced in the red marrow of the reticular tissues. When these tissues undergo pimelosis and turn yellow, the process of blood production ceases.

Bones are composed of water, organic colloidal materials, and inorganic cal-cium. Since they contain little calcium, in early walking stages, soft, infant bones often bow or bend in abnormal ways. The amount of calcium in the bones of elderly people, on the other hand, is so great that the bones are fragile and brit-tle. To correct bends in the legs of small children, improve digestion by shiatsu pressure on the abdomen and legs and in this way strengthen the bones. Taking sun baths while undergoing shiatsu therapy improves the effect by allowing the skin to absorb vitamin D from sunlight.

Functioning

1. Motion in various directions and at many angles made possible by tendons connecting bones.
2. Support of the body and preservation of normal posture (especially in the case of the spinal column).
3. Formation of body cavities—cranial cavity, spinal cavity, thoracic cavity, pelvic cavity—and protection of internal organs.
4. Production of red and white blood corpuscles and blood platelets in the marrow.
5. Storage of calcium in the osseous matter for release into the bloodstream when needed.

Joint Construction

Two bones coming together at a joint fit in the following way: the epiphysis of one is convex (convex articular surface); that of the other is concave (glenoid cavity). The joint is surrounded by the joint capsule, which forms the joint cavity. The inner membrane of the joint capsule (synovial membrane) secretes synovial fluid for the sake of lubrication. To strengthen the joint and prevent excessive extension, ligaments connect the two bones outside of the synovial membrane. Parts of these ligaments extend into the joint cavity.

Fig. 10   Joints

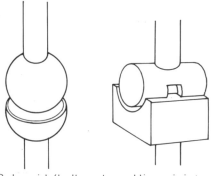

Spheroid (ball-and-socket) joint   Hinge joint (ginglymus)

Kinds of Joints

1. *Spheroid (ball-and-socket) joint.* The convex articular surface is a sphere; the concave one is a shallow cup. The shoul-der joint is an example of this kind, which is multiaxial and permits free movement through the widest range of angles. A deep glenoid cavity—like the one found in the hip joint—is characteristic of the ball-and-socket subdivision of this joint type.

2. *Hinge joint (ginglymus).* The convex articular surface is roughly cylindrical; and its axis, which is at right angles to its dia-physis, fits into the groove of the glenoid cavity of the other member forming the

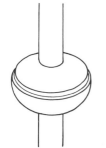
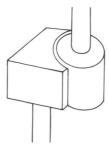

Condyloid (ellipsoid) joint   Pivot (trochoid) joint

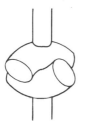
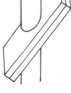

Saddle joint   Gliding joint (arthrodia)

joint. Motion of such joints is uniaxial. The interphalangeal joint is an example.

3. *Condyloid (ellipsoid) joint.* Both convex articular surface and glenoid cavity are elliptical. Such joints turn biaxially on the major and minor axes of the ellipse of the convex articular surface. The radiocarpal joint is an example.

4. *Pivot (trochoid) joint.* A cylindrical convex articular surface fits into a groove in the glenoid cavity of the other member forming the joint. Movement is possible only in the major axis of the convex articular surface. The upper radioulnar joint is an example.

5. *Saddle joint.* Convex articular surface and glenoid cavity join in a saddlelike form. Movement is biaxial, each member rotating at right angles to the other. The first carpometacarpal joint is an example.

6. *Gliding joint (arthrodia).* Since both articular surfaces are flat, movement in joints of this kind is slight: the two bones can do no more than slide parallel to each other. The intervertebral joints are of this kind.

7. *Amphiarthrosis.* The joining is achieved through small, narrow convexities and concavities; and the joints are thoroughly surrounded by tough ligaments making movement virtually impossible. The sacroiliac joint and the intercarpal joints are examples.

Fig. 11   Ossification of the Ligaments

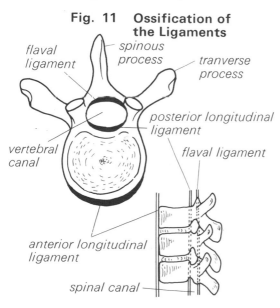

flaval ligament   spinous process   tranverse process

posterior longitudinal ligament

vertebral canal   flaval ligament

anterior longitudinal ligament

spinal canal

Irregularities in Bones and Ligaments

1. *Osteomalacia.* Primarily as a consequence of insufficient vitamin D, bones—especially the long bones—suffer a shortage of calcium and soften. Unusual bends to the front, rear, or side in the spinal column, O- or X-type bends in the legs, and deformations of the thorax are caused by this disease.

2. *Ossification of the longitudinal ligaments.* Connective ligaments are attached to the front and rear parts of the vertebrae (see Fig. 11). When some of them ossify as a result of histological changes in the bones —especially the posterior longitudinal ligaments, which face the spinal cord—the spinal column is constricted with resultant bodily impairment. The flaval ligaments on

the rear part of the spinal cord tend, not to ossify, but to become hypertrophic because of induration of the erector spinae muscles. This condition restricts movement, impairs blood circulation, reduces metabolism, and constricts the spinal cord.

3. *Bone porosis*. This symptom of aging results in reduced calcium in the osseous tissues, thinning of the dense layer of the bone, expansion of the marrow cavities, and consequent brittleness and weakness that cause bones to break easily and can result in curvature.

Fig. 12   Normal Range of Motions

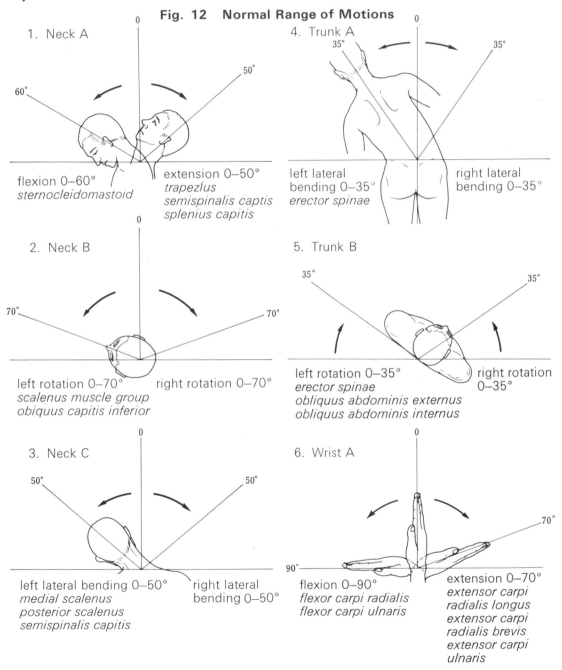

1. Neck A

0

50°

60°

flexion 0–60°
sternocleidomastoid

extension 0–50°
trapezius
semispinalis captis
splenius capitis

2. Neck B

0

70°   70°

left rotation 0–70°
scalenus muscle group
obiquus capitis inferior

right rotation 0–70°

3. Neck C

0

50°   50°

left lateral bending 0–50°
medial scalenus
posterior scalenus
semispinalis capitis

right lateral bending 0–50°

4. Trunk A

0

35°   35°

left lateral bending 0–35°
erector spinae

right lateral bending 0–35°

5. Trunk B

35°   35°

left rotation 0–35°
erector spinae
obliquus abdominis externus
obliquus abdominis internus

right rotation 0–35°

6. Wrist A

0

70°

90°

flexion 0–90°
flexor carpi radialis
flexor carpi ulnaris

extension 0–70°
extensor carpi radialis longus
extensor carpi radialis brevis
extensor carpi ulnaris

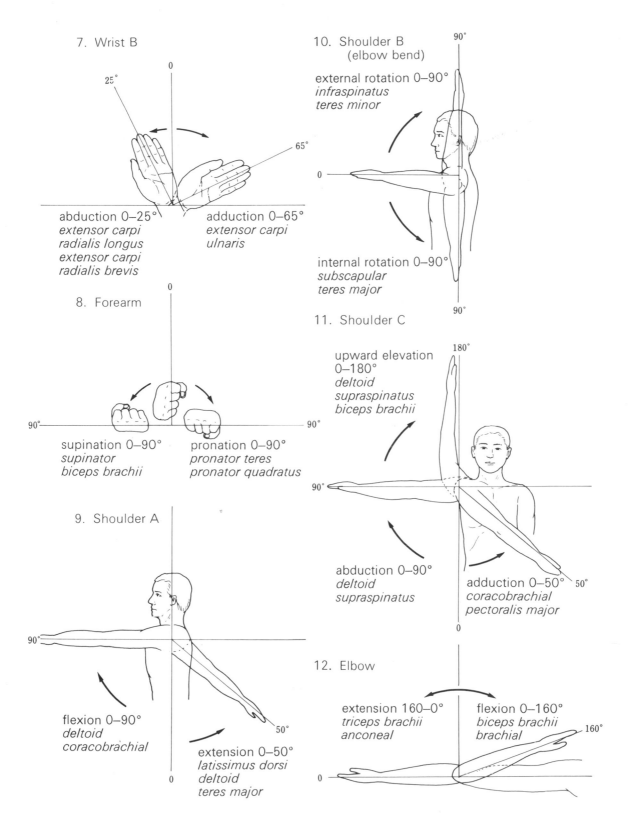

7. Wrist B

abduction 0–25°
*extensor carpi
radialis longus
extensor carpi
radialis brevis*

adduction 0–65°
*extensor carpi
ulnaris*

8. Forearm

supination 0–90°
*supinator
biceps brachii*

pronation 0–90°
*pronator teres
pronator quadratus*

9. Shoulder A

flexion 0–90°
*deltoid
coracobrachial*

extension 0–50°
*latissimus dorsi
deltoid
teres major*

10. Shoulder B
(elbow bend)

external rotation 0–90°
*infraspinatus
teres minor*

internal rotation 0–90°
*subscapular
teres major*

11. Shoulder C

upward elevation
0–180°
*deltoid
supraspinatus
biceps brachii*

abduction 0–90°
*deltoid
supraspinatus*

adduction 0–50°
*coracobrachial
pectoralis major*

12. Elbow

extension 160–0°
*triceps brachii
anconeal*

flexion 0–160°
*biceps brachii
brachial*

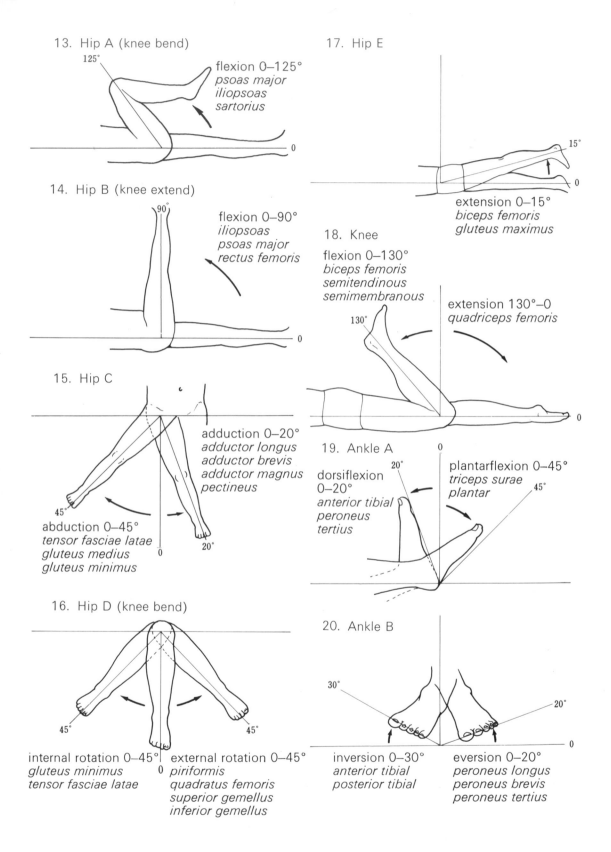

13. Hip A (knee bend)

125°

flexion 0–125°
psoas major
iliopsoas
sartorius

0

14. Hip B (knee extend)

90°

flexion 0–90°
iliopsoas
psoas major
rectus femoris

0

15. Hip C

adduction 0–20°
adductor longus
adductor brevis
adductor magnus
pectineus

45°

20°

abduction 0–45°
tensor fasciae latae
gluteus medius
gluteus minimus

0

16. Hip D (knee bend)

45°   45°

internal rotation 0–45°   external rotation 0–45°
gluteus minimus   0   *piriformis*
tensor fasciae latae   *quadratus femoris*
                             superior gemellus
                             inferior gemellus

17. Hip E

15°

0

extension 0–15°
biceps femoris
gluteus maximus

18. Knee

flexion 0–130°
biceps femoris
semitendinous
semimembranous

extension 130°–0
quadriceps femoris

130°

0

19. Ankle A

0

dorsiflexion
0–20°
anterior tibial
peroneus
tertius

20°

plantarflexion 0–45°
triceps surae
plantar

45°

20. Ankle B

30°

20°

inversion 0–30°
anterior tibial
posterior tibial

eversion 0–20°
peroneus longus
peroneus brevis
peroneus tertius

0

7. Alimentary System

Oral Cavity

The flavor and taste of food put into the oral cavity stimulate the secretion of saliva. Mastication is the action whereby the combined movements of tongue, lips, and upper and lower jaws crush food and mix it with saliva to facilitate movement into the esophagus. The process is a combination of mechanical (mastication) and chemical (saliva) actions.

Saliva is always being secreted, but tastes and odors of food increase its output volume. This is generally a nonconditioned reflex, though associations of sight or smell of foods with which one is familiar stimulate saliva secretion on the basis of a condition reflex. The salivary gland consists mainly of the parotid

Fig. 13 Passage of Food and Air   **Fig. 14 Model Drawing of the Alimentary System**

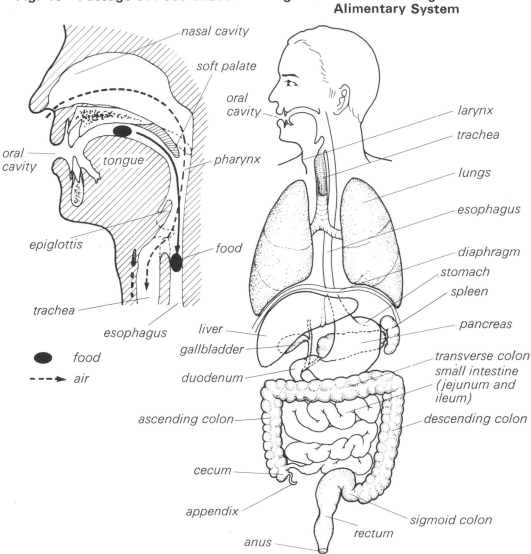

gland, the submaxilliary gland, and the sublingual gland. Ordinarily, these glands secrete from 1 to 1.5 liters of saliva daily. Saliva contains a glycoprotein called mucin, which, when mixed with food facilitates mastication and swallowing. The digestive ferment, ptyalin, in saliva breaks down starches and converts them into maltose; this is why rice that has been chewed for a long time gradually comes to taste sweet. Parotin, the hormone secreted by the parotid gland and present in saliva, is intimately connected with metabolism in bones, teeth, and connective tissues and is related to blood plasma and the reproductive system.

Pharynx

When preparations are made in the oral cavity for food to pass into the esophagus, a series of muscular contractions occurs. The soft palate blocks the nasal cavity, the larynx is raised, the epiglottis is pressed against the root of the tongue, and thus the trachea is blocked, allowing the food to pass into the esophagus in the process called swallowing.

Esophagus

The upper part of the esophagus, a tube about twenty-five centimeters long, is composed of striated muscles; the lower part is of smooth muscle. As a result of an action called peristalsis, food passes through the esophagus into the stomach in a few seconds. Liquids pass instantaneously.

Stomach

With a volume capacity of from 1.5 to 2 liters, the stomach is the largest organ in the alimentary system. The entrance from the esophagus into the stomach is called the cardia; the exit from the stomach into the duodenum is called the pylorus. The stomach is generally oriented to the left side of the body. The cardia is forward and to the right of the eleventh thoracic vertebra, and the pylorus is to the front and right of the first lumbar vertebra. The stomach lining secretes gastric juice, containing hydrochloric acid, the proteolytic enzyme pepsin, and so on. Though gastric juice plays the major role in the digestion of food in the stomach, its secretion is stimulated by the secretion of gastrin from the mucous lining of the pylorus. For food to be reduced to semifluid chyme in the stomach requires about two or three hours. Peristalsis gradually moves semifluid chyme to the pylorus and from there into the small intestine. The secretion of mucous protects the wall of the stomach from the powerful digestive actions of pepsin. But, when, stress or some other trouble obstructs blood circulation to the stomach and sufficient mucous is not secreted, the lining itself may undergo digestion. Peptic ulcers are the result of this condition.

Small Intestine

The intestines, consisting of the large intestine, small intestine, and rectum, extract a maximum of the nutrients from the chyme transported from the stomach. The small intestine consists of the duodenum, jejunum, and ileum. Absorption of required materials from chyme is practically completed in the duodenum. When foods enters this part of the intestine, hormone action stimulates the secretion of mildly alkaline bile and pancreatic fluid, which neutralize the powerful acidity of the gastric juice in the chyme. Enzymes in the pancreatic fluid and intestinal juices break down nutrients. Bile assists in this process by facilitating emulsification of fats.

The chyme next passes into the jejunum, where villi attached to the intestinal walls, which is several times thicker than the skin, absorb nutrients. Finger-shaped villi contract and expand with the movement of the smooth muscles of the intestines. Fats are carried to the lymph spaces in the villi. The other nutrients move then from the capillaries to portal veins and the liver, and then to the greater circulation through the veins. The fats move from small lymph spaces to larger ones and finally to the thoracic duct, the main canal of the lymphatic system. Lymph can then move to the abdominal cavity, upward to the vein under the left clavicle, through the upper major vein, and to the right atrium of the heart. By means of these processes, nutrients absorbed from the small intestine are circulated throughout the body.

Large Intestine

The large intestine, which is made up of the cecum, colon, and rectum, is a long (1.5 meter), thick vessel into which passes the content of the small intestine. By this time most of the nutrients in the chyme have already been absorbed, and the content of the large intestine is usually highly liquid and contains undigested, unabsorbed materials and leftover digestive juice. At the point of juncture between the large and small intestines is the appendix, which, when inflamed, causes the sickness known as appendicitis. The material in the large intestine moves from the ascending colon to the transverse colon and the descending colon and from there to the sigmoid colon. Transportation from part to part of the system is controlled by valves. As it moves along the intestine, the content is made semi-solid by reduction of liquids. As it halts for a time in the sigmoid colon, further liquid is removed, producing normal feces, which are moved by peristalsis into the rectum. Involuntary contraction of the rectum walls and relaxation of the anal sphincters remove feces from the body. Peristalsis in the large intestine is often especially strong after breakfast. Unless peristalsis operates normally, feces are not transported in an orderly fashion from the sigmoid colon to the rectum; and constipation results. Shiatsu therapy regulates the absorption of nutrients in the intestine and the process of digestion.

Operations of the Hands and Fingers

In development from primitive stages to the technologically sophisticated civilization of today, man has relied strongly on his hands. Together with powers of thought and ratiocination, the superb motor abilities of the hands and fingers distinguish man from the other animals. Human hands have made possible the acquisistion of all manner of techniques from the simple ones of scooping water to drink and plucking food to eat to the evolution of tools for striking fire, cultivation and storage of food, and hunting. Manually rubbing, pressing, and stroking parts of the body that are in pain are some of the uses to which these remarkable organs have long been put. Other animals who lack the mobile human hand must lick their bodies to cure wounds or flex their total covering or cutaneous muscles to rid themselves of pesky insects that man brushes away with his hands. (Except for the mimic muscles of the face and the platysma of the anterior cervical region, the human body generally lacks cutaneous muscles.)

Though the apes, man's closest relatives, have five-fingered hands, since their thumbs are less well developed, their hands are clumsier. The human thumb is equipped with a complex consisting of eight muscles that makes it opposable to the other fingers and that enables it to rotate. In infants this complex is undeveloped, and dexterity is limited until both intellect and the hands improve with advancing age.

Construction of the Hands and Fingers

The hairless palms of the hands lack sebaceous glands but are covered with fine curve-and-whorl patterns (Fig. 15) consisting of the cristae and sulci cutis, which are composed of connective tissues. There are sweat pores in the cristae cutis. These patterns account for the great sensitivity of the palms and make it easy to grip or hold things without their slipping from the hands.

The so-called tactile elevation at the digital ball, interdigital ball, thenar (radial carpal ball), and hypothenar (ulnar carpal ball) are highly sensitive. Among them, the tactile elevation of the thumb and index and ring fingers are most sensitive. In shiatsu therapy, thermally sensitive elements in these tactile elevations enable the therapist to judge the warmth or coolness of the patient's skin. Meissner's corpuscles provide tactile sensations; Ruffini's corpuscles, sensations of heat; Paccinian corpuscles, sensations of pressure; Krause's corpuscles, sensations of cold; and free nerve endings, sensations of pain. All of these are of the greatest importance in enabling the shiatsu therapist to judge hardness of the flesh and body temperature. The more experienced the person, the softer and more supple his hands, and the greater his ability to evaluate even subtle physical changes on the basis of touch alone.

Fingernails

The nails are modified horny substances in the skin surface that take the form of thin, horny plates. One end of the nail body is the free edge; the other, the nail root,

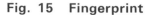

Fig. 15   Fingerprint

sulci cutis

sweat pore

cristae cutis

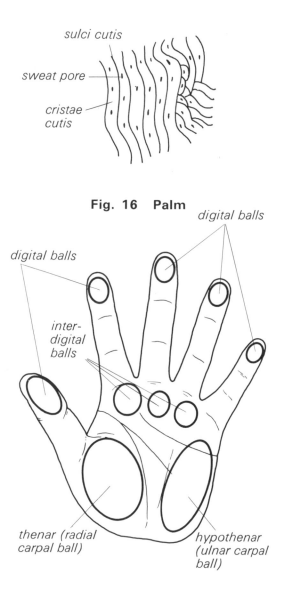

Fig. 16   Palm

digital balls

digital balls

inter-
digital
balls

thenar (radial carpal ball)

hypothenar (ulnar carpal ball)

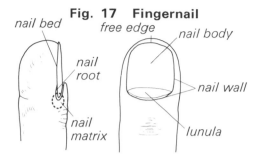

Fig. 17 Fingernail

nail bed

free edge

nail body

nail root

nail wall

nail matrix

lunula

arises from the skin of the finger. The underside of the nail, which consists of a germinative layer and cutis, is called the nail bed. The inner layer of the skin where the nail bed begins is called the nail matrix; it is here that growth of the nails (from 0.1 to 0.14 millimeters daily) takes place. The whitish crescent at the base of the nail—the lunula—is freshly produced nail substance that has not completely hardened.

Abnormalities

1. *Reedy nails.* A nail marked by longitudinal furrows is caused by neural-related malnutrition, insufficient vitamin A, or artificial stimulus (like that of acetone or fingernail polish).

2. *Spoon nails,* a condition in which the central portion of the nail is depressed. This is caused by duodenal hook worms, eczema, or insufficient iron in the blood.

3. *Hippocratic nails,* a condition in which the ends of the nails cover the tip of the finger and the nail walls, is caused by obesity in the fingertips and thickening of the nail bed and is associated with lung ailments, bronchial illnesses, hereditary heart conditions, and cyanosis.

Five Basic Rules for Good Health and Long Life

Combining an orderly, regulated way of life with observation of the five rules outlined below and regular shiatsu will help make life longer and more pleasant.

Proper Diet

Eating as much of everything you like is a diet that must be corrected. No matter how wholesome the foods you eat, balance must be maintained among them. First of all, it is essential to ensure enough of the three major energy foods—proteins, fats, and carbohydrates—to facilitate an active life. In addition, the required amounts of minerals, water, and various vitamins needed to break down these foods and convert them into energy must be included in the diet.

Even with balanced menus, the body must be able to digest and assimilate the nutrients it takes in. Ensure that this is possible by eating at regular times in proper quantities and by chewing your food well. Breakfast is a must, even if it is only a small amount of highly nutritive food. Furthermore, the connection between the organs of digestion and the vagus nerves means that emotional stress can cause upsets in the alimentary system. Avoid this by eating slowly and in a pleasant, calm atmosphere. This is all the more important since worry and irritation disrupt the functioning of the other internal organs as well.

Shiatsu on the abdomen (see p. 116) improves the functioning of the stomach and intestines, thus stimulating digestion and absorption of nutrients. It may be self-administered.

Proper Sleep

Human beings sleep about one-third of their lives if they take eight full hours of rest nightly. Sufficient sleep is more essential to recovery from fatigue than any therapy or drug. No matter how static one remains, as long as the body is awake, the organs continue to function; and the muscles preserve a state of tension. In sleep, however, the organs and the cerebral nerves rest; and the muscle relax, enabling the body to recover from weariness and be refreshed upon awakening.

There are many sleep patterns. The ideal one is falling asleep shortly after retiring, dropping into deep sleep soon thereafter, and remaining in deep sleep until sleep gradually becomes increasingly shallow and waking occurs. This process can be compared to an aircraft that takes off, immediately gains flight altitude, remains on altitude for the majority of the trip, and gradually descends to land again at the destination point.

It is said that, though they are often forgotten, everyone has dreams every night. The level of sleep in which dreams occur is the rapid-eye-movement state, which is less desirable than deep sleep. Overindulgence in alcohol results in a sleeping state that is only half sleep and half intoxication. Since he does not enjoy restful, deep sleep, the person who has drunk too much often suffers from the state known as hangover on the morning after.

There is no doubt that "early to bed and early to rise" are linked with longevity. But the tempo of modern urban living makes it difficult to follow the sound advice inherent in these words. Nonetheless, it is good to get up early in the morning and enjoy clean air before the pollution of daytime traffic has a chance to sully it. For a vigorous way of life, combine deep breathing of fresh morning air with a balanced diet, sound sleep, plenty of fresh air, and regularly administered shiatsu.

Proper Elimination

Normally the bowels should move once a day, often immediately after breakfast. If this regimen is regularly observed, the alimentary system will function correctly; and nutrients will be readily absorbed.

The amount and nature of foods eaten determine the kinds and quantities of feces eliminated. Excess consumption of difficult-to-digest foods causes either constipation or diarrhea. Psychological states too influence elimination.

To stay in good condition, eat a balanced diet regularly and perform self-administered abdominal shiatsu (p. 116) each morning. Upon waking, while lying on our back, press slowly on each of the points shown for from three to five seconds. Pressure should be applied with the palm of one hand. The other hand should be placed on top of the pressing hand. Repeat this as many times as seems necessary and then apply careful shiatsu pressure with three fingers to the area of the sigmoid colon to prevent constipation. Repeated daily, this therapy will restore appetite, improve digestion, and regulate elimination. It will help prevent constipation in people who are inclined to this condition.

Proper Exercise

One of the most direct ways to prompt good health is proper energetic exercise combining leisure, work, and sports or some other active recreation. Human beings find a reason for living in purposeful, goal-oriented activity; but in today's mechanized society, opportunities to display vitality are becoming increasing limited. Work is now subdivided and automated to the extent that human beings frequently do nothing but monotonous, repetitive operations. Means of transportation have become so convenient that people use their legs less than they should and prefer an elevator or escalator to even a moderate flight of steps. Under these conditions, it is scarcely surprising that people do not get enough exercise and that their muscular vigor declines. Recently, jogging has become popular with those who want to supplement their exercise or loose weight. But, without going this far, it is possible to achieve good results merely by walking more and moving the body as much as possible in ordinary daily activities. Walking is especially good, since it activates circulation in the legs and relieves sluggishness that inactivity causes. In addition, it is important to make full use of the bending, stretching, reaching, and lifting that are parts of the movements performed in many apparently minor daily tasks.

From the shiatsu standpoint, I recommend special attention to exercising the hands and fingers. Small children who do not exercise these parts of the body enough fail to develop reflexes that could prevent injury in falls. Moving the hands and fingers develops the motor nerves that stimulate self-protective reflex extensions of the hands and arms. I recommend encouraging children in the lower grades of primary school to administer shiatsu to themselves regularly. The shiatsu designed to strengthen the eyes and teeth (p. 161) is especially good since hand and finger exercises of this kind are related to cerebral functioning. The hand motions involved in painting, writing, playing the piano, or craft work have a good influence on powers of thought.

Laughter

Laughter is unique to the human being. A naturally laughing face is pleasing and beautiful. Physiologically, laughter is healthful and improves the color of blood. In contrast, anger and fear cause the face to become livid and create pathological tensions in the internal organs. The up-down movement of the diaphragm caused by laughter stimulates the operation of the heart, improves the circulation, and activates the functioning of the stomach and intestines. In addition, it helps regulate the internal secretions of the endocrine system. Illness makes truly beautiful laughter difficult or impossible.

Mimic muscles—risorius and major zygomatic muscles—at the ends of the mouth produce the smile and the facial expression of laughter. Stroking this area on the faces of infants causes them to smile in their own innocent, natural way. The artificial, forced smile that people sometimes wear is always wry and unpleasant.

A good guffaw from the bottom of the belly once a day contributes to a better way of life. As the old sayings have it, "Laughter is the gate to happiness" and "A laugh rejuvenates, a frown ages."

Fig. 18   A Laugh Rejuvenates; a Frowns Ages

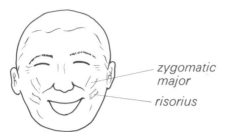

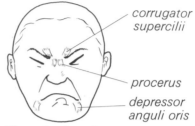

corrugator
supercilii

zygomatic
major

risorius

procerus

depressor
anguli oris

*When the face smiles the
stomach smiles too.*

*When the face frowns, the
stomach frowns too.*

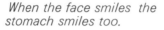

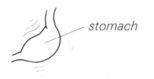

stomach

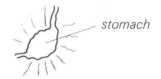

stomach

Conditions Requiring Shiatsu Therapy

Head
Headache, migraine, heaviness in the head, insomnia, neuroses, alopecia areata, occipital neuralgia, malnutrition of the hair and scalp

Face
Temporary myopia, hyperopia, strabismus, ptosis, asthenopia, blockage of the nose, sinusitis, tic paralysis, trigeminal neuralgia, toothache, alveolar blennor-rhea, facial paralysis, roughness of the skin

Anterior cervical region
Heart disease, insomnia, toothache, cerebral anemia, dizziness, congenital myogenic torticollis, whiplash syndrome, arteriosclerosis, climacteric upsets, autonomic imbalance, hiccoughs, dysthyroidea, chorditis

Lateral cervical region
Whiplash syndrome, arteriosclerosis, migraine, dizziness, tinnitus, hardness of hearing, motion sickness

Medulla oblongata
Whiplash syndrome, nosebleed, heaviness of the head, headaches, neuroses, insomnia, autonomic imbalance, dizziness on standing, climateric upsets

Posterior cervical region
Insomnia, arteriosclerosis, headaches, migraine, occipital neuralgia, whiplash syndrome

Suprascapular region
Stiff shoulders, scapulohumeral perarthritis, loss of appetite, heartburn, brachial neuralgia

(left side) Heart disease, upsets of the stomach and abdomen, pancreatic illness
(right side) Gastroptosis, liver complaints, gallstones

Interscapular region

Bronchial asthma, respiratory illness, heartburn, intercostal neuralgia, loss of appetite, scoliosis in the thoracic vertebrae
(left side) Upsets of the stomach and intestines, pancreatic ailments, heart disease
(right side) Liver ailments, gallstones

Infrascapular region

Diabetes, kidney complaints, malfunctioning of the suprarenal bodies, constipation, diarrhea, lumbago, hernia of the intervertebral discs, sciatica, lordosis, kyphosis, scoliosis, nocturnal enuresis
(left side) Upsets of the stomach and intestines, pancreatic ailments
(right side) Liver complaints, gallstones

Iliac crest

Constipation, intestinal disorders, chilling, accumulation of subcutaneous fat, diarrhea, lumbago

Sacral region

Prostate complaints, illness of the bladder, irregular menstruation, impotence, nocturnal enuresis, frigidity, obstruction in secretion of sex hormones

Gluteal region

Sciatica, chilling, fatigue in the legs, hemorrhoids, frigidity

Namikoshi points

Diarrhea, constipation, sciatica, lumbago, fatigue in the legs, hernia of the intervertebral discs, irregular menstruation, menstrual pains, chilling, gallbladder complaints, impotence, hypertrophy of the prostate gland, nocturnal enuresis, frigidity, premature ejaculation

Legs

Sciatica, fatigue in the legs, chilling, pains in the knees, edema of the legs, beriberi, cramps in the gastrocnemius muscle, contraction of the Achilles' tendon, kidney complaints, hemiplegia, nocturnal enuresis, articular rheumatism, SMON disease, dislocation of the hip joint, bowlegs, knock-knees, talipes valgus, talipes varus, talipes equinus, talipes calcaneus, contraction of the quadriceps femoris muscle

Arms

Scapulohumeral perarthritis, brachial neuralgia, paralysis of the median nerve, paralysis of the radial nerve, paralysis of the ulnar nerve, articular rheumatism, hemiplegia, Raynaud's disease, writer's cramp
(inner side of the left upper arm) Heart disease

Chest region

Bronchial asthma, intercostal neuralgia, insufficient lactation
(left side) Heart disease

Abdominal region

Loss of appetite, gastrospasm, gastroptosis, heartburn, yawning, liver ailments, constipation, diarrhea, diabetes, gastroatony, gastric hyperacidity, gallstones, chilling, menstrual pains, irregular menstruation, insomnia, high blood pressure, low blood pressure, arteriosclerosis, nocturnal enuresis, agenesia, gastritis, nervous stomachache, obesity, impotence

Conditions for Which Shiatsu Therapy MUST NOT BE APPLIED

1. Contagious illnesses
2. Pleurisy, peritonitis, appendicitis, pyelitis, pancreatitis, peptic ulcers, duodenal ulcers, liver cirrhosis, leukemia, twisting of the bowels, intestinal obstruction, cancer
3. High fever immediately after surgery, extreme physical debility, infectious skin ailments

Points of Caution

1. The hands must be clean and the fingernails cut to a suitable length at all times.
2. Before begining treatment, the therapist must breathe deeply to regulate respiration and unify himself mentally.
3. The basics of correct therapy must be mastered.
4. Proper basic positions for therapy must be mastered. If the positions are not maintained carefully, pressure will not be stabilized as it should.
5. Pressure points must be accurately located. From the outset, pressure must be of the correct intensity. It must never be too great.
6. When the patient suffers from a condition making it impossible to move the body freely—scapulohumeral perarthritis, sprains, pregnancy, hernia of the intervertebral discs, whiplash syndrome, hemiplegia, and so on—the therapist must take special care to adjust himself to the patient's positions and regulate intensity of pressure application.
7. During therapy, the therapist must concentrate on his work with sincerity and caution.
8. Therapeutical sessions should last from thirty minutes to one hour, depending on the age, sex, condition, and symptoms of the patient.
9. The patient should urinate or defecate if necessary before therapy begins and should relax physically and mentally. Of course, if it is essential, therapy can be stopped midway.
10. Therapy sessions should begin no sooner than thirty minutes after meals, when the stomach is neither empty nor too full.

Chapter 2

Basic Operations

Kinds of Pressure Application

1. Thumb Pressure

As is seen in Fig. 1, composed of only the proximal and distal phalanges and lacking the middle phalanx found in the other fingers, the thumb is short and thick. Stability plus well-developed digital ball and well-attached musculature make the thumb the most widely used finger in shiatsu therapy. It can operate with considerable strength over a wide range. Furthermore, the great area of the fleshy ball (where the finger-print is located) makes possible wider distribution of skin sense organs and consequent increase in sense-receptor powers.

Some people's thumbs naturally bend well at the distal phalanx—soft type (Fig. 2); the thumbs of other people do not—hard type (Fig. 3). In shiatsu, pressure is applied with the digital ball of the thumb. In the case of the soft type, the pressure must not be applied with the joint between the distal and proximal phalanges (interphalangeal joint); and in the hard type, it must not be applied with the tip of the thumb. In the first instance, full application of the digital ball produces pleasurable sensations in the patient; in the second, sharper and more stimulating sensations. As the therapist develops skill, he will learn when to use the soft pleasurable pressure and when—as, for example, in cases of paralysis and muscular hardening—to apply the sharper pressure of the digital ball of the thumb.

Fig. 1 Correct Way to Apply Pressure with the Thumb

The joint between the metacarpal bone and proximal phalanx (metacarpophalangeal joint) is slightly bent. When this point is tensed, pressure may be applied with the digital ball of the thumb.

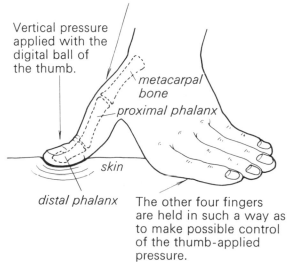

Vertical pressure applied with the digital ball of the thumb.

metacarpal bone

proximal phalanx

skin

distal phalanx

The other four fingers are held in such a way as to make possible control of the thumb-applied pressure.

Fig. 2 Soft type

Do not press with the interphalangeal joint.

interphalangeal joint

Fig. 3 Hard type

Do not press with the tip.

tip of distal phalanx

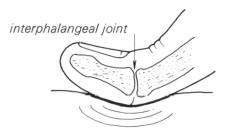

Fig. 4   One-thumb Pressure

One-thumb Pressure

Pressure is applied with the thumb of either the right or the left hand, and the four fingers are placed lightly on the patient's body as support (Fig. 4).

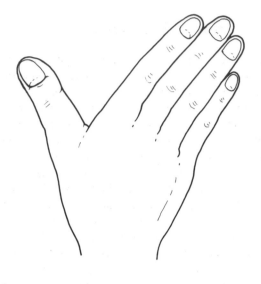

Fig. 5   Two-thumb Pressure

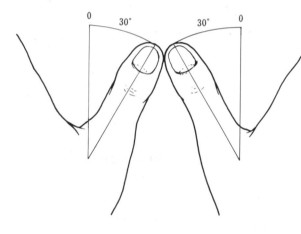

Two-thumb Pressure

The thumbs of both hands are brought together so that their outer edges touch slightly and so that each thumb is open to about thirty degrees (Fig. 5). The other four fingers of each hand are held together. Pressure is applied with both thumbs simultaneously.

Fig. 6   Thumb-on-thumb Pressure

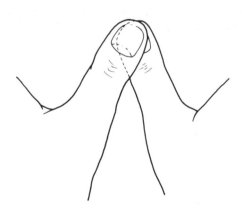

Thumb-on-thumb Pressure

The digital ball of the left thumb is placed lightly on the nail of the right thumb (reverse for left-handed people), and each thumb is open to about thirty degrees, as in two-thumb pressure applications. With the right thumb fixed firmly in place, pressure is applied at the same time with both (Fig. 6). Too much force should not be applied with the thumb on top, and load should not be put on the thumb underneath.

2.   Two-digit Pressure

Pressure with Opposed Thumb and Index Finger

Holding the digital ball of the thumb and that of the index finger of the same hand about as far apart as shown in Fig. 7, the therapist applies pressure with both. This is used in applications of pressure to the fingers and toes.

Pressure with Middle and Index Fingers

The digital ball of the middle finger is placed on the fingernail of the index finger of the same hand. This finger position (Fig. 8) makes possible stable pressure application with the digital ball of the index finger. It is used in shiatsu on the sides of the nose.

Fig. 7   Pressure with Opposed Thumb and Index Finger

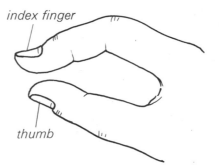

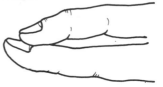

index finger

thumb

Fig. 8   Pressure with Middle and Index Fingers

Fig. 9   Pressure with Left Middle Finger on Right Middle Finger

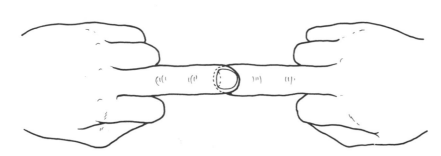

Pressure with Left Middle Finger on Right Middle Finger

The digital ball of the left middle finger is placed on the fingernail of the right middle finger. Stable pressure is applied with both (Fig. 9). (Finger positions are reversed for left-handed people.) This finger position may be used in self-administered shiatsu on the medulla oblongata.

Pressure with Open Index and Middle Fingers

The middle and index fingers of the same hand are opened to the angle shown in Fig. 10. Pressure is applied simultaneously with both. This finger position is used in treating both sides of the spinal column of small infants.

Fig. 10   Pressure with Open Index and Middle Fingers

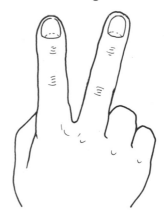

3. Three-finger Pressure

Holding them close together, press simultaneously with the index, middle, and ring fingers of the same hand (Fig. 11). This finger position is used in palpation and in self-administered shiatsu to a single point.

4. Pressure with Open Thumb and Four Fingers

The thumb and four fingers of the same hand, all oriented in the same direction and held together with a slight opening between the thumb and the other four, are used to apply pressure simultaneously (Fig. 12). This finger position is used in treating the occipital, sural, and lateral cervical regions.

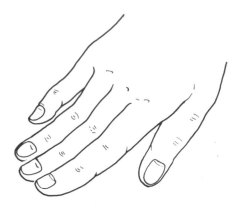

Fig. 11   Three-finger Pressure

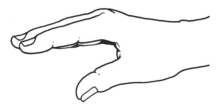

Fig. 12   Pressure with Open Thumb and Four Fingers

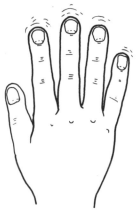

Fig. 13   Pressure with Four Fingers Held Open

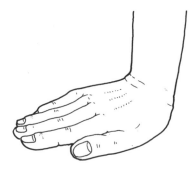

Fig. 14   One-palm Pressure

5. Pressure with Four Fingers Held Open

Pressure is applied with the four fingers—held in an open position (Fig. 13) without the assistance of the thumb. This position is used in treating the chest and intercostal region and in some kinds of self-administered shiatsu.

6. Palm Pressure

Pressure is applied with the whole palm and with the thenar (radial carpal ball) and the hypothenar (ulnar carpal ball), and the carpal region.

One-palm Pressure
All five fingers are held together, and pressure is applied with the whole palm of one hand only (Fig. 14).

Fig. 15   Hand-on-hand Palm Pressure

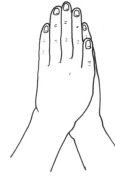

Fig. 16   Hand-on-hand (crossed) Pressure

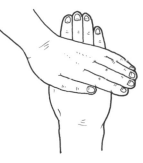

Fig. 17   Two-palm Pressure

Hand-on-hand (Crossed) Pressure

Fingers of both hands are held together firmly, and the palm of the left hand is placed on the back of the right hand (Fig. 15). A variation of this position calls for placing the palm of the left hand crosswise on the back of the right hand at right angles (Fig. 16).

Two-palm Pressure

The hands are held flat and parallel with the outer edges of the thumbs touching (Fig. 17), and pressure is exerted with both hands simultaneously. This position is used in applying undulation pressure, rotational pressure, and vibrational pressure to the abdomen.

Joined-hands Pressure

Firmly interlocking the fingers, the therapist applies pressure simultaneously with both carpal regions (Fig. 18). This position is used in applying pressure in the area of the kidneys.

Pressure with the Thenar (Radial Carpal Ball)

Pressure is applied with this part of the hand (Fig. 19) to the abdomen and the inguinal region with one hand. The same parts of both hands are used to apply pressure to the anterior superior iliac spine.

Pressure with the Hypothenar (Ulnar Carpal Ball)

In treating the abdomen, pressure is sometimes applied with the hypothenar (Fig. 19).

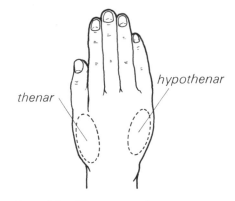

thenar   *hypothenar*

Fig. 19   Thenar and hypothenar Pressure

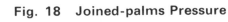

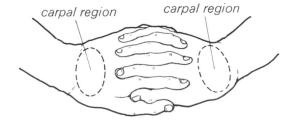

carpal region   *carpal region*

Fig. 18   Joined-palms Pressure

Kinds of Pressure

1.   Standard Pressure

In this the most widely used method, pressure is applied gently and gradually and is then gradually decreased. Application is one-phase and lasts from three to five seconds (Fig. 20).

2.   Interrupted Pressure

Operating on one point, the therapist first applies light pressure. Then, without removing the thumb (or other part of the hand being used) from the patient's skin, he relaxes pressure. Then he applies pressure of medium intensity. If the application stops here, it is two-phase. There is a three-phase version in which pressure is relaxed after the second phase and then stronger pressure is applied. Each application lasts for from five to seven seconds.

Fig. 20   Standard Pressure

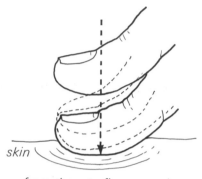
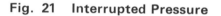

from three to five seconds

Fig. 21   Interrupted Pressure

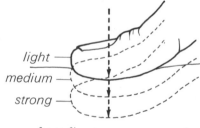

from five to seven seconds

Fig. 22   Sustained Pressure

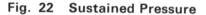
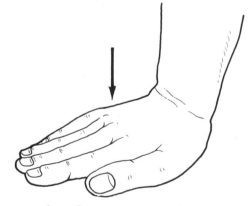

from five to ten seconds

3.   Sustained Pressure

Generally performed with the palm, this application is one-phase. The same pressure is maintained for from five to ten seconds (Fig. 22).

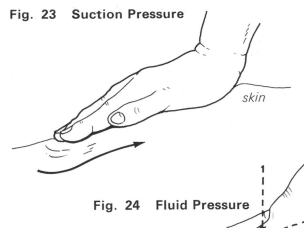

Fig. 23   Suction Pressure

4.   Suction Pressure

This very special application method, usually employing three fingers or the palm pressed well against the patient's skin, is a backward-pulling motion that seems to draw the connective tissues away from the skin (Fig. 23). Undulation pressure and rotational pressure applied to the abdomen are of this kind.

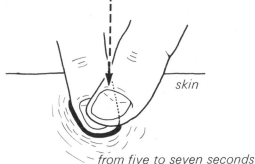

Fig. 24   Fluid Pressure

skin

from one to to two seconds

5.   Fluid Pressure

With the thumbs of the right and left hands, alternation applications of pressure lasting from one to two seconds per point are made in a succession of points either beside each other or above or below each other (Fig. 24). The transition from point to point is natural and smooth; hence the name *fluid pressure*.

6.   Concentrated Pressure

Gradually increasing pressure is applied in concentration on one spot for from five to seven seconds. When the desired intensity is reached, pressure is gradually relaxed without allowing the thumb to leave the patient's skin, then gradually increased again. The application, which may be repeated several times, is made with thumb-on-thumb pressure.

7.   Vibrational Pressure

Steady pressure is applied to the skin with the thumbs, three fingers, or the palm on a single point for from five to ten seconds. The therapist's hand vibrates throughout the application (Fig. 26). Several variations are possible: one-hand application, two-palm application, and palm-on-palm application. The pleasurable sensations that penetrate the skin of the patient make this a special kind of pressure application.

Fig. 25   Concentrated Pressure

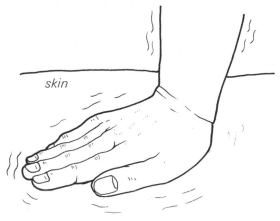

skin

from five to seven seconds

Fig. 26   Vibrational Pressure

skin

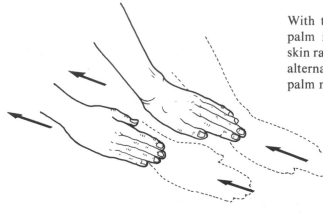

Fig. 27   Palm-stimulation Pressure

8.   Palm-stimulation Pressure

With the fingers held close together, the entire palm is pulled downward across the patient's skin rapidly (Fig. 27). Both palms may be used in alternation in quick downward motions, or one palm may be placed on the other.

Stages of Pressure Intensity

Touch
Used in palpation and diagnosis, this method calls for barely pressing the finger against the patient's skin. Maximum pressure is no more than one hundred grams.

Slight Pressure
From the touch stage, the finger moves to a very slight application of pressure and then returns at once to the touch stage. This kind of pressure is applied several times to the same point or from place to place. Intensity ranges between one hundred grams and one kilogram.

Light Pressure
Though greater than slight pressure, light pressure is still gentle. The therapist must synchronize steadily slowly increasing pressure with his own breathing. When the maximum for this intensity is reached, he must gradually relax pressure. Intensity ranges between one kilogram and five kilograms

Medium Pressure
Though, at first, pressure applications of this intensity may cause the patient slight discomfort, he will gradually come to find the sensation they produce pleasurable. Intensity ranges from five to fifteen kilograms.

Strong Pressure
Though the strongest pressure applied in shiatsu, this stage does not exceed an intensity of from fifteen to thirty kilograms. It should never cause the patient unpleasant sensations, although it may produce the kind of moderate pain that is describable as pleasant. The therapist must learn to control and sustain pressure that produces such pleasurable pain.

Fig. 28   Stages of Pressure Intensity

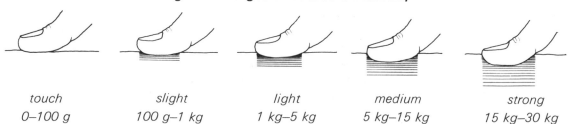

| touch | slight | light | medium | strong |
| 0–100 g | 100 g–1 kg | 1 kg–5 kg | 5 kg–15 kg | 15 kg–30 kg |

Chapter 3

Total-body Therapy

Shiatsu for a Patient Lying in the Lateral Position

The therapist must always begin this therapy with the left side. The patient lies in the right lateral position, with the right leg straight. For the sake of stability in the trunk, the left leg is crossed over the right one; and the left knee and anterior crural region lie on the floor. The trunk must lean forward to form an angle of about 60 degrees with the floor. The following explanations pertain to the left side. When therapy is completed, the patient should assume the left lateral position; and the therapist should repeat the treatment on the right side.

Cervical Region

Operation 1: Anterior Cervical Region

The therapist assumes a position behind the patient's back with left knee on the floor and right knee raised. He puts his left palm on the floor in front of the patient's chest to support his body

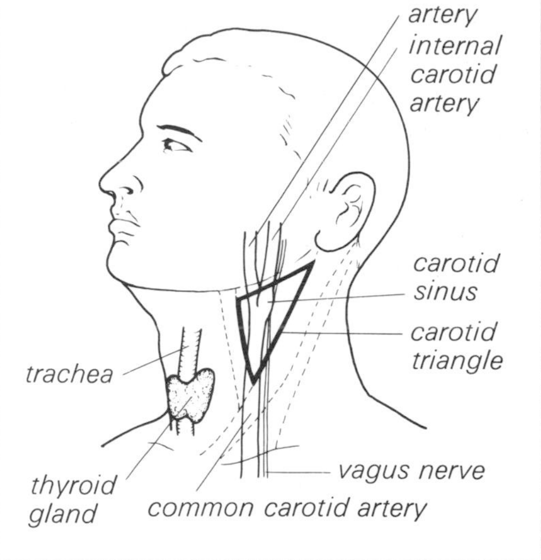

Fig. 2 Four Points in the Anterior Cervical Region

carotid triangle

Fig. 1 Carotid Sinus

external carotid artery
internal carotid artery
carotid sinus
carotid triangle
vagus nerve
trachea
thyroid gland
common carotid artery

Fig. 3

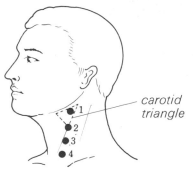

(Fig. 3). He presses his right thumb lightly against anterior cervical (front of the neck) point 1 in the carotid sinus (Figs. 1 and 2) to ascertain pulse. Taking care that they do not strike the patient's face, he brings the four fingers of his right hand to the upper part of the lateral cervical region (side of the neck) so that thumbs and hands together grip the neck lightly.

Pressure, which is not strong, but gentle, is directed toward the spinous processes of the cervical vertebrae; and the motion is made as if with a pull in the direction of the inner side of the

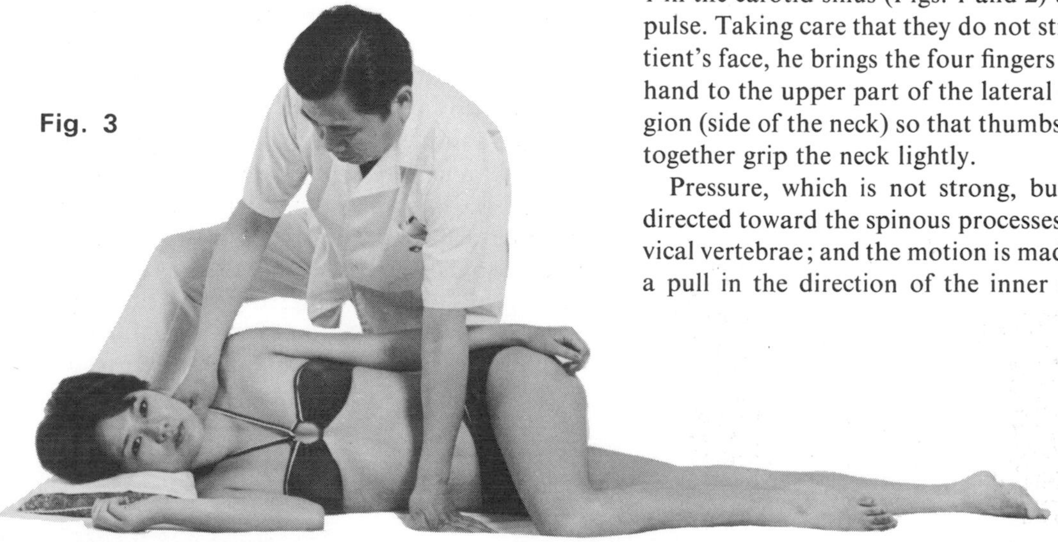

Fig. 4 Muscles and Pressure Points in the Anterior Cervical Region

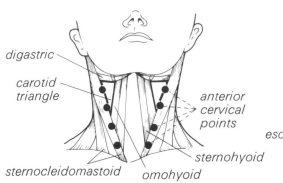

digastric

carotid triangle

anterior cervical points

sternocleidomastoid

sternohyoid

omohyoid

Fig. 5 Pressure Application on the Anterior Cervical Region

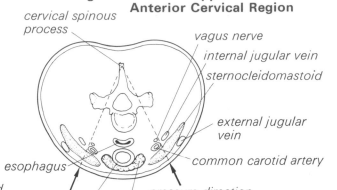

cervical spinous process

vagus nerve

internal jugular vein

sternocleidomastoid

external jugular vein

esophagus

common carotid artery

trachea

pressure direction

thyroid gland

Fig. 6

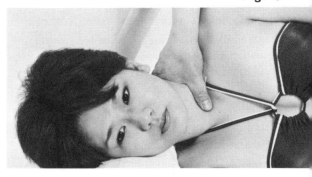

sternocleidomastoid muscle (Fig. 5). Pressure lasts for three seconds on each point. The treatment continues for all four of the anterior cervical points leading along the inner border of the sternocleidomastoid muscle to a point just before the clavicle (Figs. 2 and 4) and is repeated three times.

Fig. 7 Points in the Lateral Cervical Region

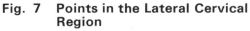

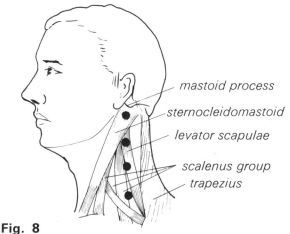

mastoid process

sternocleidomastoid

levator scapulae

scalenus group

trapezius

Fig. 8

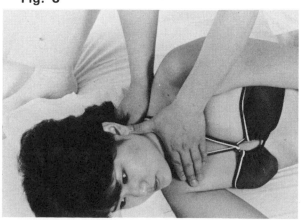

Operation 2: Lateral Cervical Region

Remaining in the same position and placing his right thumb as shown in Fig. 7, the therapist begins treatment with the first point in the left lateral cervical region, which is located directly below the mastoid process. Pressure is applied with thumb on thumb (left thumb on the nail of the right thumb, or reverse for left-handed people) and must be directed at right angles to the surface of the patient's skin (Fig. 8). Each application lasts for three seconds. All four of the lateral cervical points, which begin at 1 and continue down the cervix to the base of the shoulder and the suprascapular region, are treated in the same way. Treatment is repeated three times. Since thumb-on-thumb pressure is applied in the vertical direction with all of the therapist's weight, applications tend to be strong. For this reason, the strength of pressure must be gauged according to the condition of the part of the patient's body being treated and must never be too great.

Operation 3: Medulla Oblongata

The central part of the indentation called the nuchal fossa, which is located directly below the external occipital protuberance, is where the medulla oblongata is found (Fig. 9). To treat this area, the therapist assumes the position prescribed for operation 2. Lightly supporting the patient's forehead with the palm of the right hand, he places his left thumb, directed upward, on the medulla-oblongata region (Fig. 11) and supports the patient's right lateral cervical region with the remaining four fingers of his right hand. Pressure on one point lasts for five seconds and is directed toward the eyebrows (Fig. 10). This is repeated three times. When such therapy is applied to a patient in the lateral position, a pillow is placed under his head to prevent its moving.

Operation 4: Posterior Cervical Region

Assuming the position prescribed for operation 3, the therapist puts his right thumb at the first point of the left posterior cervical region, left of the medulla oblongata (Fig. 9). He puts his left thumb on top of his right thumb and applies pressure with both thumbs for three seconds. The pressure should be directed toward the opposite side toward the median line of the face (Fig. 12). Pressure is then applied to posterior cervical points 2, 3, and 4 in a line gradually approaching the fourth lateral cervical point (Figs. 13 through 16). This is repeated three times.

Fig. 9 Medulla Oblongata and Four Posterior Cervical Points

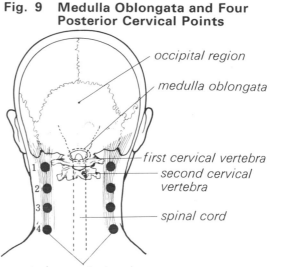

occipital region
medulla oblongata
first cervical vertebra
second cervical vertebra
spinal cord
posterior cervical region

Fig. 10 Pressure Application for the Medulla Oblongata (arrow)

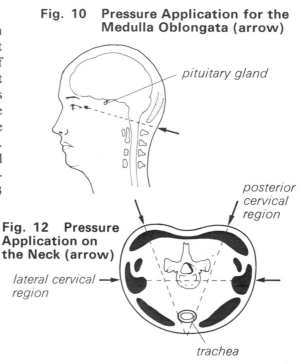

pituitary gland
posterior cervical region
lateral cervical region
trachea

Fig. 12 Pressure Application on the Neck (arrow)

Fig. 11

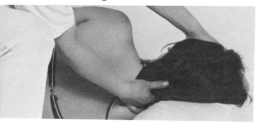

Fig. 13

Fig. 14

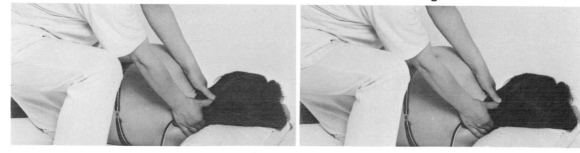

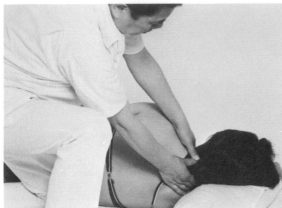

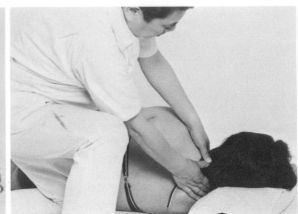

Fig. 15   Fig. 16

Back

Operation 5: Suprascapualr Region

The patient lies in the same position (Fig. 17). The therapist moves around to the crown of the patient's head and, with his left knee raised and his right knee on the floor, assumes a position fairly close to the patient's head. Extending both arms fully, he supports the patient's shoulder with the four fingers of each hand. With right thumb on left thumb, using both, he applies pressure to the suprascapular point (Figs. 18 through 20). The left thumb is on the bottom this time because, if the right one were in that position, the little-finger side of the right hand might touch the patient's face. If no such danger exists, it is permissible to put the left thumb on the right one. Pressure is directed to the center of the trunk at the height of the spinous process of the seventh thoracic vertebra. Pressure application on each point lasts five seconds. The pressure is repeated three times.

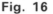

Fig. 17   Patient Posture for Treatment of the Suprascapular Point

suprascapular point

60°

Fig. 18   Pressure Direction for the Suprascapular Point (arrow)

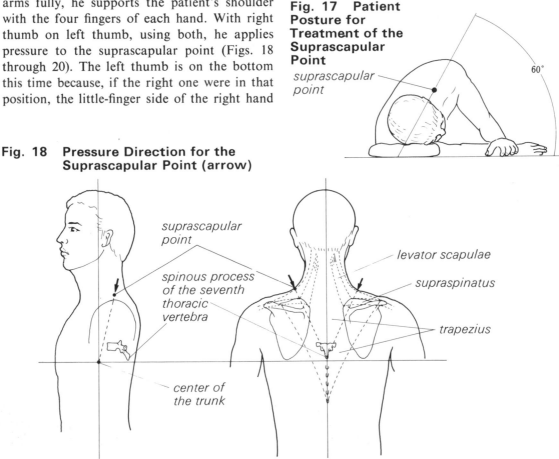

suprascapular point

spinous process of the seventh thoracic vertebra

center of the trunk

levator scapulae

supraspinatus

trapezius

Fig. 19 Treatment for the Suprascapular Point

suprascapular point

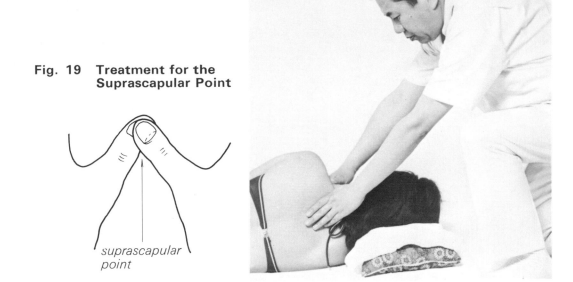

Fig. 20

Operation 6: Interscapular Region

The patient remains in the same position as in the preceding operation. The therapist moves to a kneeling position where the patient's scapulae (shoulder blades) are directly in front of him. The five points on the interscapular region (between the scapula and spinal column) run from the upper corner to the lower corner of the scapula (Fig. 21) and are parallel with the spinal column. With the right thumb on the bottom and the left thumb on the top, the therapist applies pressure for three seconds to each point, repeating three times (Fig. 22). In pressing, the trunk is held perfectly straight and slightly inclined to the front. Both arms are fully extended, and the body weight rests on the thumbs. Pressure must not be applied directly to either the scapula or the vertebrae (Fig. 23).

Fig. 21 Five Points in the Interscapular Region

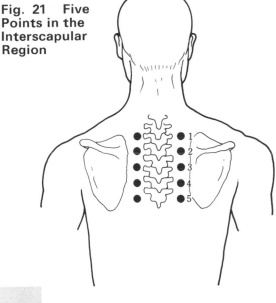

Fig. 22

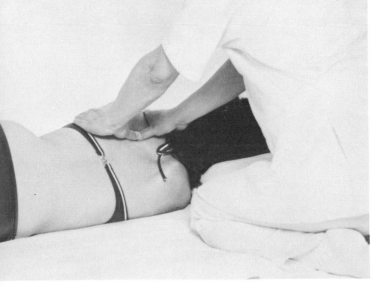

Fig. 23 Treatment for the Interscapular Region

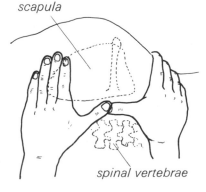

scapula

spinal vertebrae

68

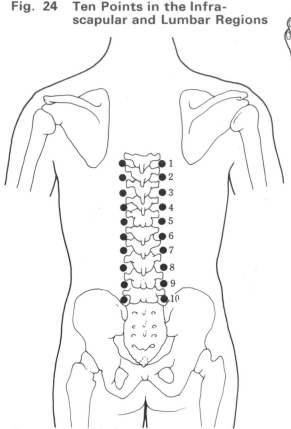

Fig. 24   Ten Points in the Infrascapular and Lumbar Regions

1
2
3
4
5
6
7
8
9
10

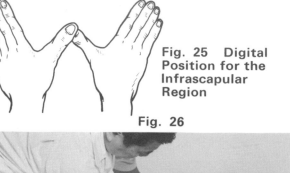

Fig. 25   Digital
Position for the
Infrascapular
Region

Fig. 26

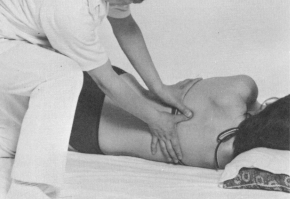

Fig. 27

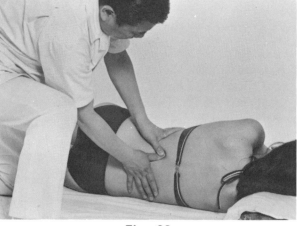

Fig. 28

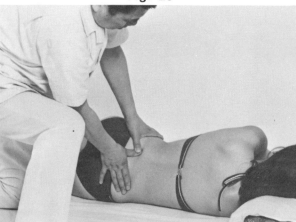

Operation 7: Infrascapular and lumbar Regions

The patient remains in the same position as in the preceding operation. The therapist moves to a position close to the patient's buttocks and kneels with left knee on the floor and right knee raised. The first point of application in this operation is the fifth point for the operation devoted to the interscapular region. The points run along the spinal column from this first point to the last, which is located between the fifth lumbar vertebra and the sacroiliac joint (Fig. 24). For the first nine points, pressure is applied for three seconds each with both thumbs—the right under the left—and is repeated three times (Figs. 25 through 28). On the last point, strong pressure is applied for five seconds in three applications.

Next, the therapist moves to a position near the patient's buttocks. Placing the left palm on the patient's buttocks, he presses the four points along the spinal column (Fig. 29), with the palm of the right hand for three seconds on each point.

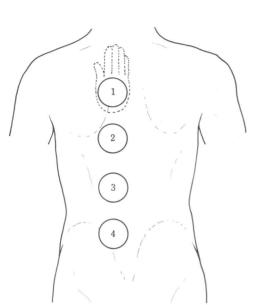

Fig. 29   Four Points for Palm Pressure on the Left Side of the Back

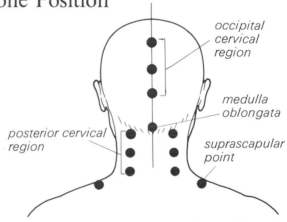

Fig. 30

This is repeated twice (Fig. 30). Finally, he strokes rapidly with the right palm all ten points from the first in the infrascapular region to the tenth in the lumbar region. This is repeated twice.

Shiatsu for a Patient in the Prone Position

Head

Operation 1: Occipital Region

The patient lies prone with head resting on a pillow and with arms straight to the sides and elbows bent upward at ninety degrees. The therapist kneels, right knee on the floor and left knee raised, by the patient's left side. With both thumbs held so that their outer edges touch each other, he presses the three points on the median line of the occipital region (Fig. 31) from the uppermost to the lowermost. Pressure is applied for three seconds to each point and is repeated three times (Fig. 32).

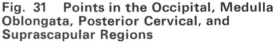

Fig. 31   Points in the Occipital, Medulla Oblongata, Posterior Cervical, and Suprascapular Regions

Fig. 32

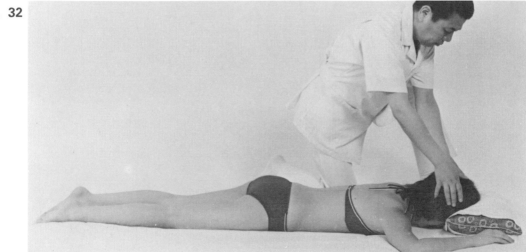

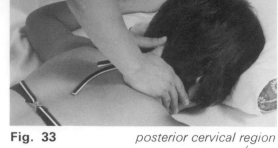

Fig. 33

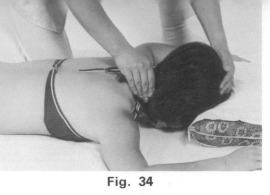

Fig. 34

Fig. 35 Treatment of the Posterior Cervical Region

posterior cervical region

Pressure exerted by thumb and four fingers must be equal.

Operation 2: Medulla Oblongata

With the right thumb on the bottom and the left thumb on top, remaining in the same position, the therapist presses the location of the medulla oblongata, slightly lower than the points in the preceding operation but directly in line with the median line (Fig. 31). Pressure lasts five seconds on each point and is repeated three times (Fig. 33).

Operation 3: Posterior Cervical Region

Remaining in the same position, the therapist applies pressure to the points in the right and left posterior cervical regions simultaneously with the thumb and four fingers of the right hand. The left hand supports the crown of the head (Fig. 34). Moving downward from the topmost of the three points, he applies pressure for three seconds on each point. The pressure should be directed through the head toward the center of the face. This is repeated three times. Pressures exerted from right and left must be equal (Fig. 35).

Shoulders and Back

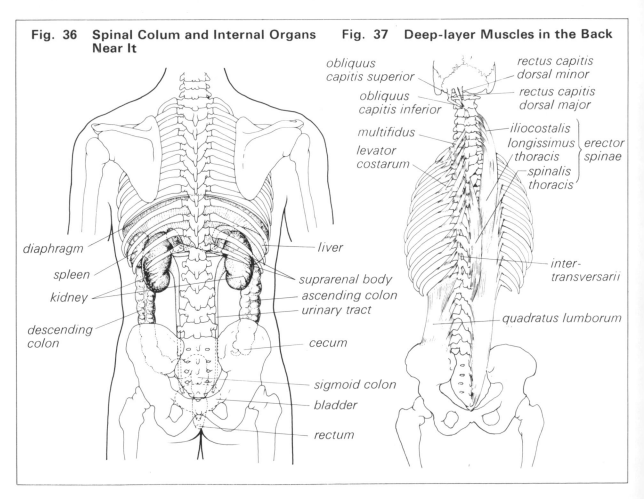

Fig. 36 Spinal Colum and Internal Organs Near It

diaphragm
spleen
kidney
descending colon
liver
suprarenal body
ascending colon
urinary tract
cecum
sigmoid colon
bladder
rectum

Fig. 37 Deep-layer Muscles in the Back

obliquus capitis superior
obliquus capitis inferior
multifidus
levator costarum
rectus capitis dorsal minor
rectus capitis dorsal major
iliocostalis
longissimus thoracis
spinalis thoracis
erector spinae
inter-transversarii
quadratus lumborum

Fig. 38 Shiatsu Points in the Spinal-column Region

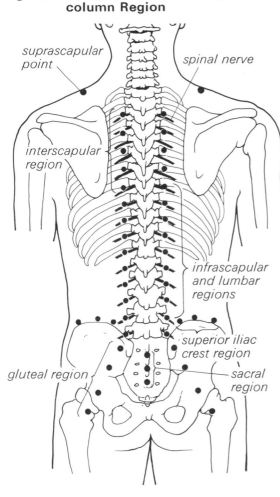

suprascapular
point

spinal nerve

interscapular
region

infrascapular
and lumbar
regions

superior iliac
crest region

gluteal region

sacral
region

Operation 4: Suprascapular Region

The patient removes the pillow and, facing left, places head and chest flat on the floor. The therapist moves to a position above the patient's head and, turning his body to a slight angle, kneels and faces the patient. Leaning well forward, he puts his right hand on the floor for support. Extending his left arm straight, he presses the left suprascapular point with the left thumb (Figs. 38 and 39). The direction of the pressure must be toward the center of the trunk at the height of the spinous process of the seventh thoracic vertebra, just as is the case in shiatsu for this point in the lateral position (Figs. 40 and 41). Pressure is applied for five seconds and repeated three times.

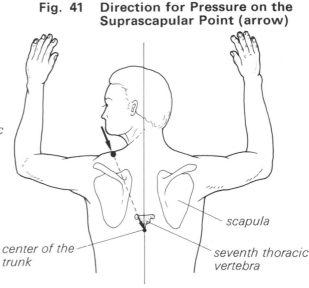

Fig. 39

Fig. 41 Direction for Pressure on the Suprascapular Point (arrow)

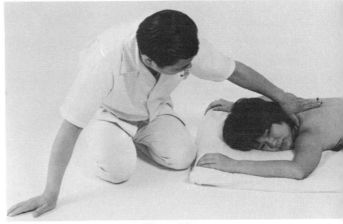

center of the
trunk

scapula

seventh thoracic
vertebra

Fig. 40 Transverse Cross Section of the Chest

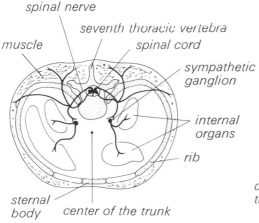

spinal nerve

seventh thoracic vertebra

muscle

spinal cord

sympathetic
ganglion

internal
organs

rib

sternal
body

center of the trunk

Fig. 42

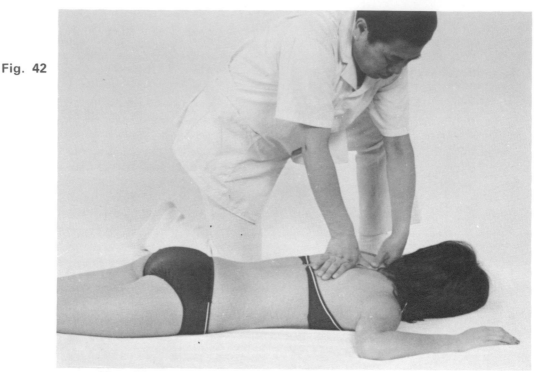

Fig. 43

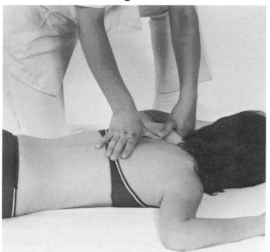

Fig. 44

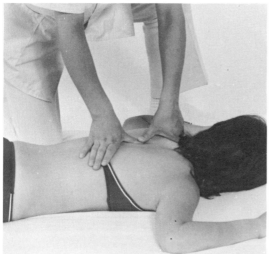

Operation 5: Interscapular Region

The patient remains in the same position as in the preceding operation. The therapist kneels, right knee on the floor and left knee raised, beside the patient's trunk on the left side and raises his hips. From this position, he extends both arms and straightens his elbows. With right thumb underneath and left thumb on top, he applies two-thumb pressure to the five points in the interscapular region parallel with the spinal column, working from the uppermost point downward (Figs. 42 through 44). His weight will be transmitted naturally through his straightened elbows. Pressure is applied for three seconds on each point and is repeated three times. Care must be taken not to press directly on either the scapula or the vertebrae, but in the area between them parallel with the spinal column; that is, on the erector spinae muscles (Fig. 45).

Fig. 45 Treatment for the Interscapular Region

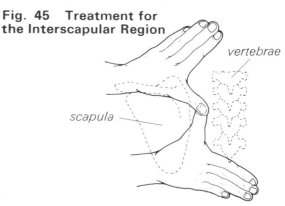

vertebrae

scapula

Fig. 46 Treatment for the Infrascapular and Lumbar Regions

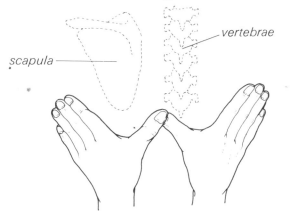

scapula

vertebrae

Operation 6: Infrascapular and Lumbar Region

Remaining in the same posture, the therapist moves downward to a position beside the patient's buttocks. Two-thumb pressure (right thumb on the bottom) is applied in this case too, but the thumb tips are pointed upward (Fig. 46). Point 5 of the interscapular region is point 1 for the infrascapular region. Pressure is applied, one by one, to the ten points from this point to the last point, which is located beside the fifth lumbar vertebra. The points are aligned parallel to the spinal column (Fig. 38). Pressure is applied for three seconds on each, and therapy is repeated three times (Figs. 47 through 50). On the third repetition, strong pressure is applied for five seconds to the tenth point and is repeated three times.

Fig. 47
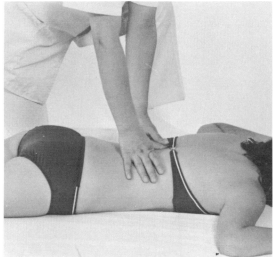

Fig. 48
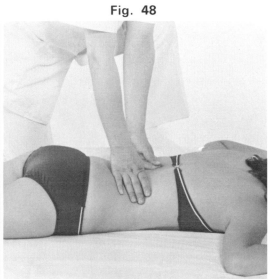

Fig. 49
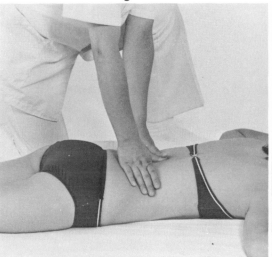

Fig. 50
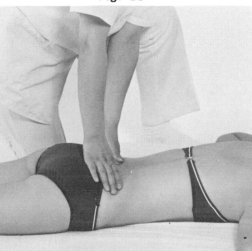

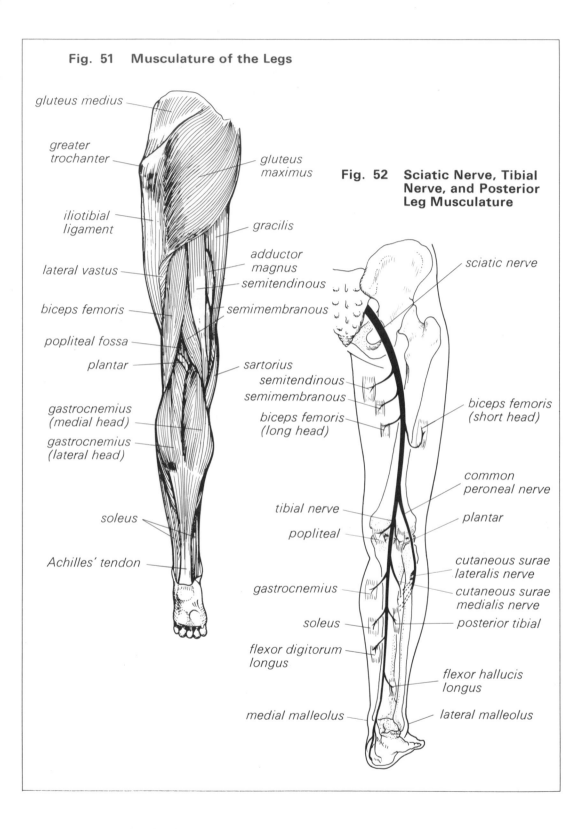

Fig. 51 Musculature of the Legs

gluteus medius

greater trochanter

iliotibial ligament

lateral vastus

biceps femoris

popliteal fossa

plantar

gastrocnemius (medial head)

gastrocnemius (lateral head)

soleus

Achilles' tendon

gluteus maximus

gracilis

adductor magnus

semitendinous

semimembranous

sartorius
semitendinous
semimembranous

biceps femoris (long head)

Fig. 52 Sciatic Nerve, Tibial Nerve, and Posterior Leg Musculature

sciatic nerve

biceps femoris (short head)

common peroneal nerve

tibial nerve

popliteal

plantar

gastrocnemius

cutaneous surae lateralis nerve

cutaneous surae medialis nerve

soleus

posterior tibial

flexor digitorum longus

flexor hallucis longus

medial malleolus

lateral malleolus

Buttocks and Legs

Operation 7: Illiac Crest

Moving still farther toward the patient's feet, using thumb-on-thumb pressure, the therapist presses the three points that lead upward along the iliac crest from the sacral region (Fig. 53). Pressure lasts for three seconds on each point, and treatment is repeated three times (Figs. 54 through 56).

Fig. 53 Shiatsu Pressure Points on the Buttocks and Posterior Legs

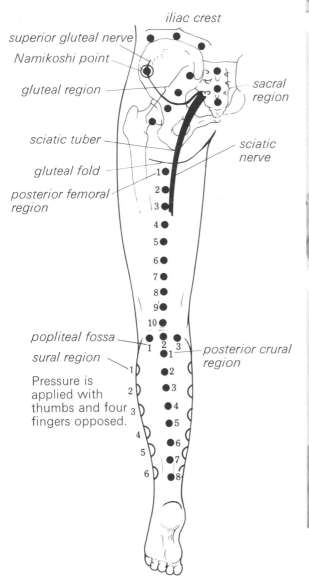

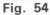

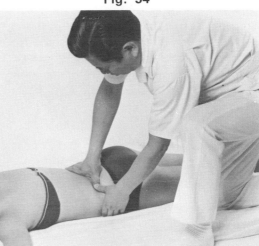

Fig. 54

Fig. 55

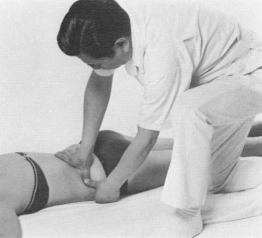

Fig. 56

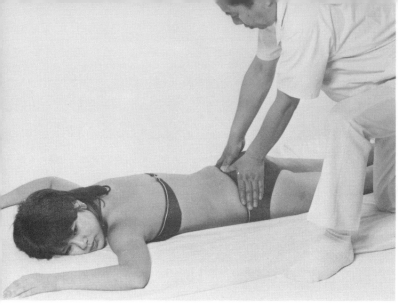

Fig. 57

Fig. 58

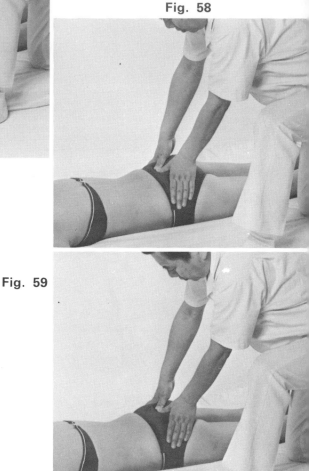

Fig. 59

Operation 8: Sacral Region

Remaining in the same position as for operation 7 and using both thumbs with their outer edges touching each other, the therapist presses three times for three seconds on each point along the median line of the sacral crest (Figs. 38 and 53). This is the region of origin of the erector spinae muscles.

Fig. 60

Fig. 61

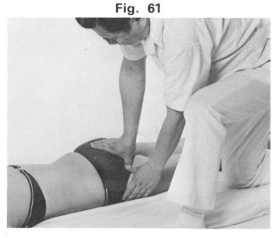

Operation 9: Gluteal Region

Placing the thumb of the right finger on the first gluteal point (Fig. 53), located immediately to the side of the first sacral-region point, the therapist puts his left thumb on top of his right thumb and presses for three seconds. Pressure is directed toward the greater trochanter. He then presses on points 2, 3, and 4 (Fig. 51), which are located on a downward slanting line across the gluteus maximus muscle (Figs. 60 and 61).

Fig. 62 The Namikoshi Point

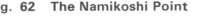

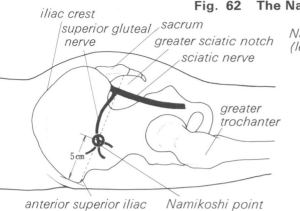

iliac crest
superior gluteal nerve
sacrum
greater sciatic notch
sciatic nerve
greater trochanter
5 cm
anterior superior iliac spine
Namikoshi point (left side)

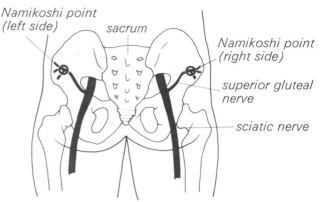

Namikoshi point (left side)
sacrum
Namikoshi point (right side)
superior gluteal nerve
sciatic nerve

Fig. 63

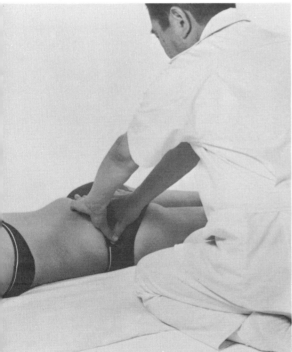

Operation 10: Namikoshi Point

The patient remains in the same position as in the preceding operation. The therapist kneels on both knees on the left side of the patient's buttocks. The Namikoshi point is located on the line connecting the anterior superior iliac spine and the sacrum, about five centimeters from the anterior superior iliac spine and near the greater sciatic notch (Fig. 62). With the right thumb underneath, strong kneading pressure is applied on this point with both thumbs for five seconds and is repeated three times (Fig. 63).

Operation 11: Posterior Femoral Region

The therapist kneels—right knee on the floor, left knee raised—by the side of the leg at the position of the popliteal fossa and turns to face the patient's thighs. The first pressure point in this region is in the gluteal fold directly below the sciatic tuber (Fig. 53). The trunk of the sciatic nerve passes through this zone. The therapist presses this point strongly three times with both thumbs, the right thumb underneath, for three seconds each. He proceeds to administer three-seconds of pressure three times to each of the ten points between the first point and the popliteal fossa.

Fig. 64   Fig. 65

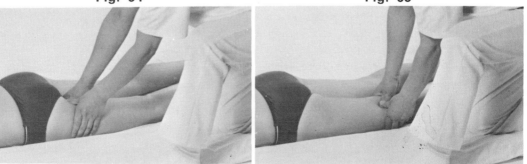

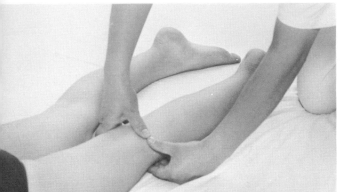

Operation 12: Popliteal Fossa

Remaining in the same posture, the therapist moves farther toward the patient's feet. With both thumbs held so that their outer edges touch each other, he applies three seconds of pressure three times to each of the three points (Fig. 53) in the popliteal fossa, moving from the outside inward (Fig. 66).

Fig. 66

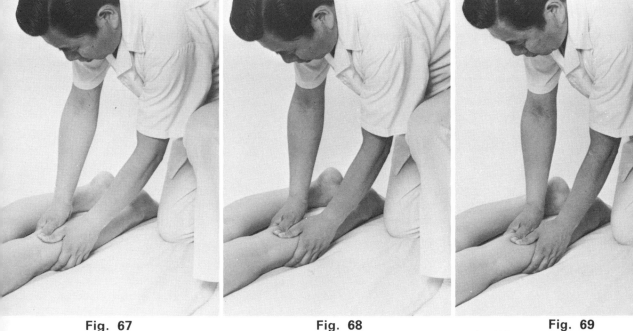

Fig. 67   **Fig. 68**   **Fig. 69**

Operation 13: Posterior Crural Region

Remaining in the same posture, moving still farther rearward, and using both thumbs, held so that their outer edges touch each other, the therapist applies three seconds of pressure three times to the eight points (Fig. 53) starting directly below the second point in the popliteal fossa (Figs. 67 through 70). These points lie along the triceps surae muscles (lateral and medial heads of the gastrocnemius muscle, and soleus muscle). Since tension in these muscles varies from person to person, pressure applications must be gauged to the individual case.

Fig. 70

Fig. 71

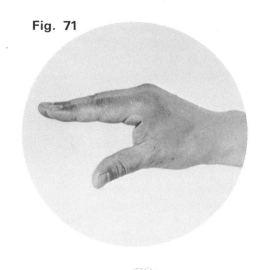

Next the therapist faces the patient's calf from the side and kneels upright on both knees. Holding the hands as shown in Fig. 71, he grips the calf and, applying squeezing pressure of a duration of three seconds, moves downward from the gastrocnemius muscle to the Achilles' tendon. Six applications are required to cover the distance. The process is repeated three times (Figs. 72 and 73).

Fig. 72

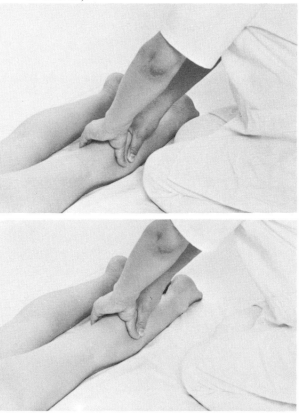

Fig. 74 Operation for the Calcaneal Tubercle

Fig. 73

Fig. 75

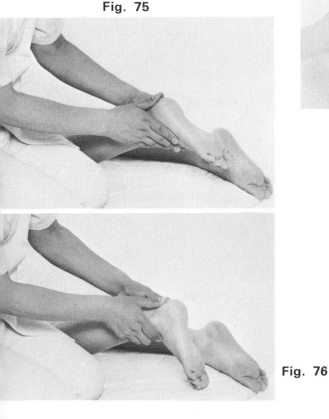

Operation 14: Calcaneal Tubercle (Extension of the Achilles' Tendon)

The therapist faces the patient's ankle joint and kneels on both knees. Putting both thumbs, held so that their outer edges touch each other, on the calcaneal tubercle and, wrapping the other fingers around the ankle for support, he lightly lifts the foot upward (Figs. 74 through 76). Holding it in this position, he applies kneading pressure to the three points on the tubercle on the side of the Achilles' tendon. The pressure lasts for three seconds on each point and is repeated three times. This treatment extends the Achilles' tendon.

Fig. 76

Fig. 77 Shiatsu Points for the Calcaneal-tubercle Region

Fig. 78 Shiatsu Points for the Sides of the Calcaneus

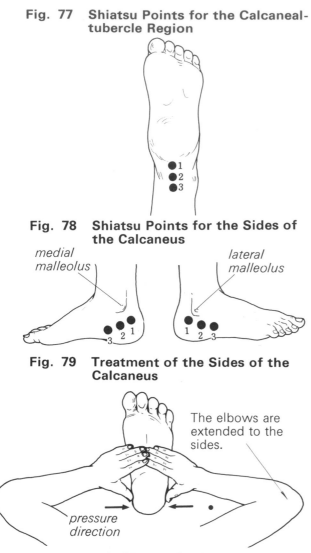

Fig. 79 Treatment of the Sides of the Calcaneus

Operation 15: Lateral and Medial Calcaneus (Malleolus) Region

Remaining in the same position and lowering the patient's foot, the therapist puts his right thumb on the first of the three points between the calcaneus bone and the lateral malleolus and his left thumb on the first of the three points between the medial malleolus and the calcaneus. The fingers of the left hand overlap with the fingers of the right hand, and both are placed on the bottom of the foot for support. Pressure is applied simultaneously to both sides on the three points (Fig. 79) in a line moving from the malleolus toward the toes. The applications last three seconds each and are repeated three times (Fig. 80).

Fig. 80

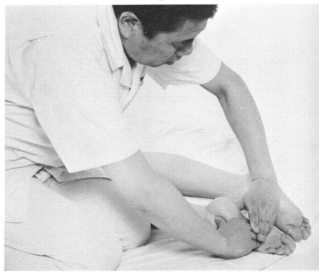

Operation 16: Plantar Region

Remaining in the same location, the therapist kneels with left knee on the floor and right knee raised. The four pressure points (Fig. 81) are located on a straight line down the middle of the sole, beginning immediately below the gap between the bases of the second and third toes and extending to the heel. Pressure is applied with both thumbs, held so that their outer edges touch each other, for three seconds each time for three times on these points (Fig. 83). The plantar arch is treated last; with the right thumb underneath, both thumbs are used to apply pressure to the point three times for five seconds each (Figs. 84 and 85).

Fig. 81 Shiatsu Points in the Plantar Region

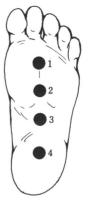

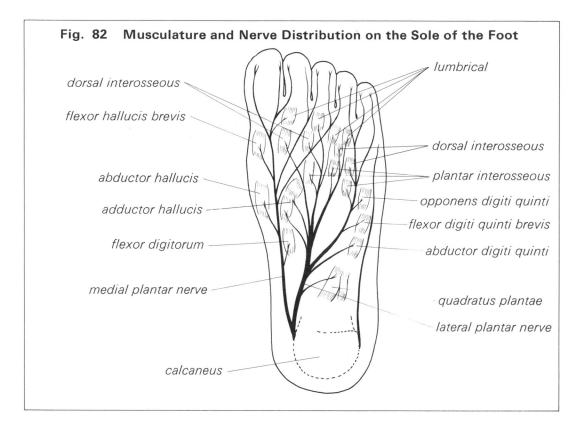

Fig. 82   Musculature and Nerve Distribution on the Sole of the Foot

lumbrical

dorsal interosseous

flexor hallucis brevis

dorsal interosseous

plantar interosseous

abductor hallucis

opponens digiti quinti

adductor hallucis

flexor digiti quinti brevis

flexor digitorum

abductor digiti quinti

medial plantar nerve

quadratus plantae

lateral plantar nerve

calcaneus

Fig. 83   Thumb Positions for Treatment of the Plantar Region

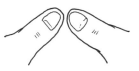

Fig. 84   Thumb-on-thumb Pressure in the Plantar Region

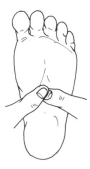

Fig. 85

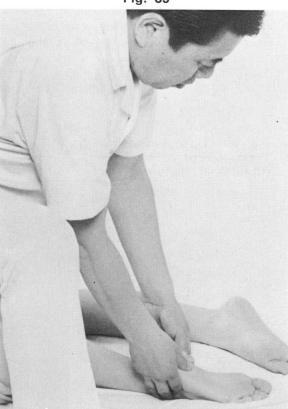

Adjusting the Back

Operation 1: Scapulae

The therapist kneels—left knee on the floor, right knee raised, and hips up—on the left side of the patient near the scapulae. With extended elbows, he places his right palm over the patient's right scapula and his left palm over the left scapula. The palms should be pressed completely and firmly against the skin. First with the left then with the right hand, the therapist executes circular rotational pressure in an outward direction; that is, clockwise with the right hand and counterclockwise with the left hand. This is done three times on each side (Fig. 86) then five times simultaneously on both scapulae (Fig. 87).

Operation 2: Lateral Abdominal Region

Moving slightly rearward, the therapist positions his hands on the both of the patient's lateral abdominal regions so that the four fingers of each press against his body at about the position of the diaphragm and the thumbs lie immediately below the scapulae and the diaphragm. Synchronizing his movements with his breathing, on the count of one, the therapist pushes upward; on the count of two, downward (Fig. 88). He repeats this rhythmically ten times (Figs. 89 and 90).

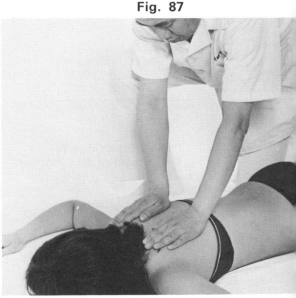

circular rotational pressure on the scapulae

circular rotational pressure on the buttocks

Fig. 86   Circular Rotational Pressure on the Scapulae and Buttocks

Fig. 87

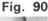

Fig. 88   Up-down Treatment of the Lateral Abdominal Region

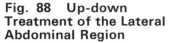

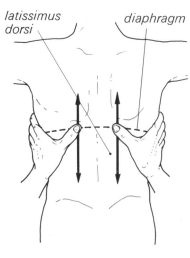

latissimus dorsi   *diaphragm*

Fig. 89   **Fig. 90**

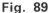

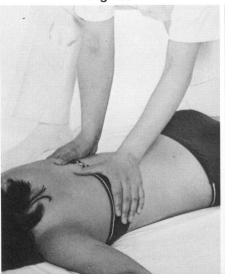

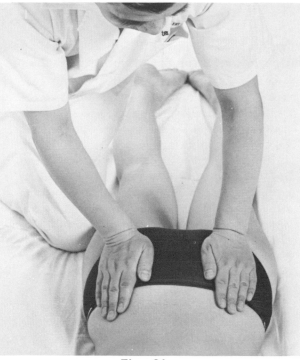

Fig. 91

Operation 3: Gluteal Region

Remaining in the same posture, the therapist slides rearward to the location of the patient's hips and places his right hand flat on the right buttock and left on the left buttock. Circular, outward-directed pressure is applied just as in the treatment of the scapulae (Fig. 86): three times on the left buttock, three times on the right buttock, and five times simultaneously on both (Fig. 91).

Operation 4: Spinal Column (Transverse Processes)

Kneeling on both knees, the therapist turns to face the patient's spinal column. Then, raising his hips, with both palms placed over the location of the spinal column (Fig. 92), he pushes up then down. The palms of both hands must be pressed firmly against the patient's body. Dividing the distance between the upper thoracic vertebra and the lumbar vertebra into six equal parts, he presses twice on each location with a rhythm of one, two, three, and four (Fig. 93). The position of the hands moves gradually down the spine throughout the operation (Figs. 94 and 95).

Fig. 92   Adjusting the Transverse Processes of the Spinal Column

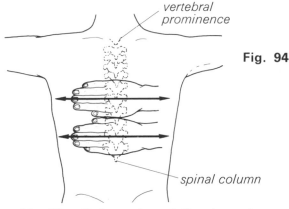

vertebral prominence

spinal column

Fig. 93   Six Points for Adjusting the Transverse Processes of the Spine and Spinous Processes

Fig. 94

Fig. 95

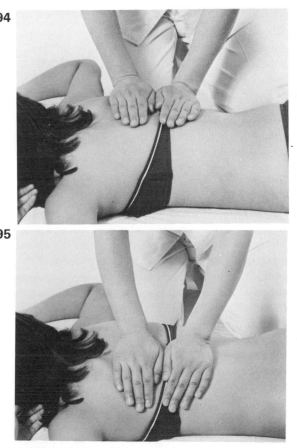

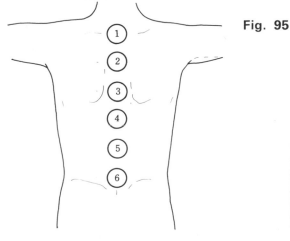

Fig. 96   Adjusting the Spinous Processes

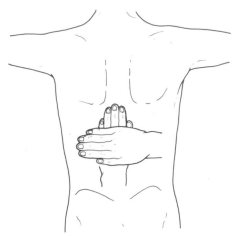

Operation 5: Spinal Column

Kneeling on the left knee with the right knee raised and hips lifted, as in operation 4, for the transverse processes, the therapist treats the spinous processes on the same six points (Fig. 93). He presses his left palm on the spinal column with fingers pointed toward the patient's head and then places the right hand across the left at ninety degrees (Fig. 96). At this time, the middle finger of the left hand must be aligned exactly with a point directly below the spine of the seventh cervical vertebra. As he presses, the therapist has the patient exhale slowly in synchronization with his pressure application. Pressure is applied for one second to each point, and the therapy is repeated twice. The therapist's hands move gradually downward during the course of treatment. Pressure must be steady, with no sharp interruptions.

Fig. 97

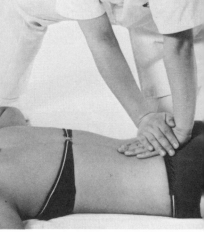

Fig. 98

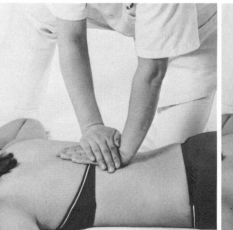

Fig. 99

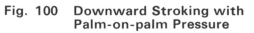

Operation 6: Stimulating the Spinal Nerves

At the conclusion of operation 5, remaining in the same position, the therapist immediately returns his left palm to a position on the spinal column directly below the spinous process of the seventh cervical vertebra, fingers pointed toward the patient's head, and puts his right hand on top of his left. The fingers of the right hand too point toward the patient's head. With both hands, he strokes rapidly all the way down the spinal column to the sacrum (Figs. 100 through 102). He repeats this three times.

Fig. 100   Downward Stroking with Palm-on-palm Pressure

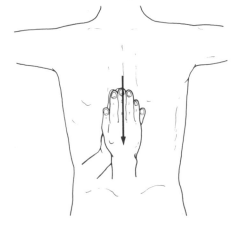

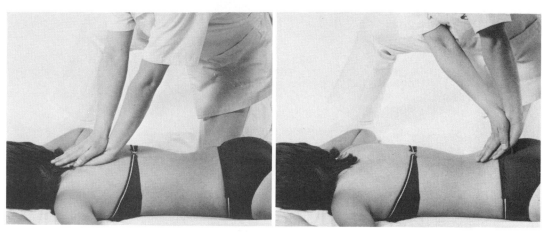

Fig. 101   Fig. 102

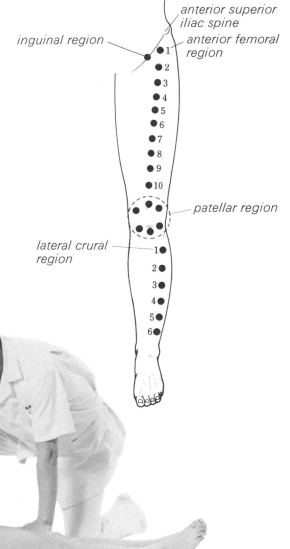

Shiatsu for a Patient Lying in the Supine Position

Legs

Operation 1: Anterior Femoral Region

The patient lies supine with head on a pillow, legs straight, and arms straight by the sides. The therapist, kneeling on the left knee with the right knee and hips raised, assumes a position on the left side of the patient, facing the thighs. He slightly presses the digital ball of his right thumb on the center of the patient's groin—a point between the anterior superior iliac spine and the pubic bone (Fig. 103). The tip of the thumb is directed slightly outward and diagonally to the right. The palm of the left hand lightly supports the lower part of the anterior femoral region immediately above the knee (Fig. 104). Pressure is applied vertically to the groin point with the right palm for five seconds and is repeated three

Fig. 103   Shiatsu Points on the Anterior Surface of the Leg

anterior superior iliac spine

inguinal region

anterior femoral region

patellar region

lateral crural region

Fig. 104

86

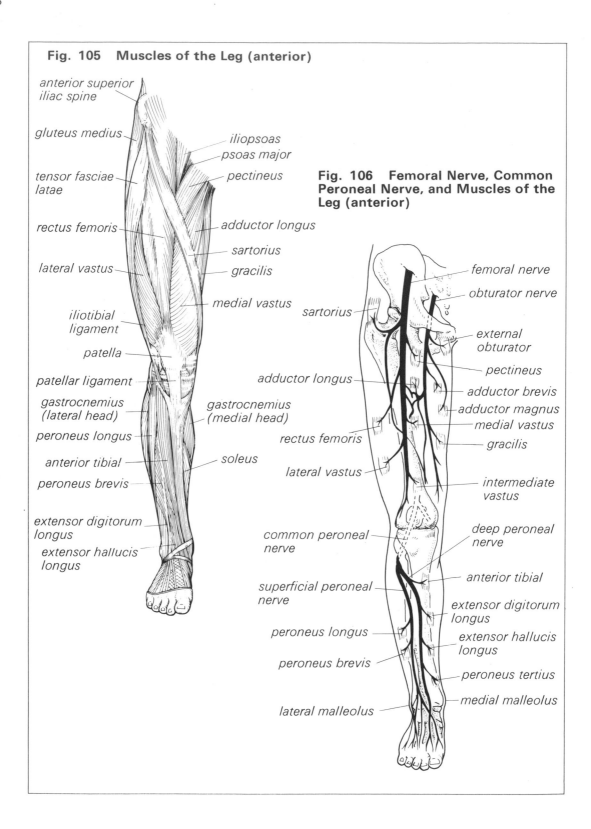

Fig. 105   Muscles of the Leg (anterior)

anterior superior iliac spine

gluteus medius

tensor fasciae latae

rectus femoris

lateral vastus

iliotibial ligament

patella

patellar ligament

gastrocnemius (lateral head)

peroneus longus

anterior tibial

peroneus brevis

extensor digitorum longus

extensor hallucis longus

iliopsoas
psoas major

pectineus

adductor longus

sartorius

gracilis

medial vastus

gastrocnemius (medial head)

soleus

Fig. 106   Femoral Nerve, Common Peroneal Nerve, and Muscles of the Leg (anterior)

sartorius

adductor longus

rectus femoris

lateral vastus

common peroneal nerve

superficial peroneal nerve

peroneus longus

peroneus brevis

lateral malleolus

femoral nerve

obturator nerve

external obturator

pectineus

adductor brevis

adductor magnus

medial vastus

gracilis

intermediate vastus

deep peroneal nerve

anterior tibial

extensor digitorum longus

extensor hallucis longus

peroneus tertius

medial malleolus

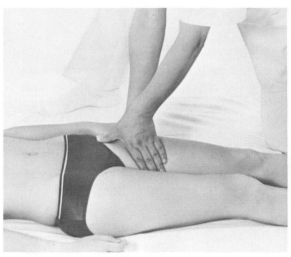

Fig. 107

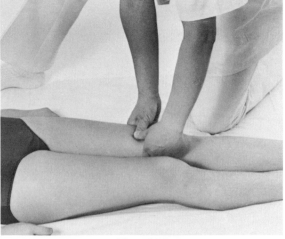

Fig. 108

times. Next, he presses with both thumbs, right thumb underneath, on the ten points (Fig. 103) from immediately below the anterior superior iliac spine to a location just above the knee joint. Pressure applications last for three seconds on each point, and the treatment is repeated three times (Figs. 107 and 108).

Operation 2: Medial Femoral Region

The therapist remains in the same position. But the patient turns the right knee outward and brings the left heel to the Achilles' tendon of the left foot (Fig. 110). With both thumbs, right thumb underneath, the therapist presses on each of the points (Fig. 111) from immediately below

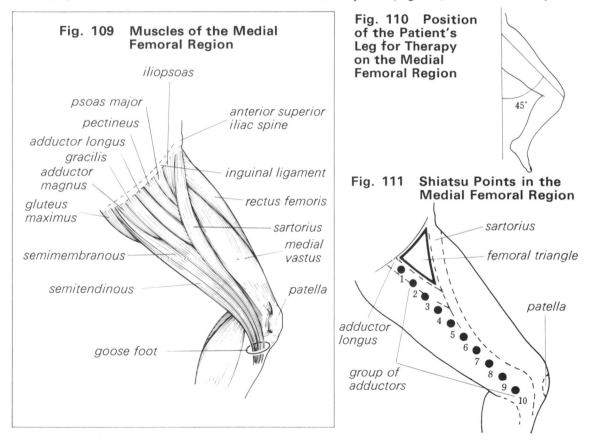

Fig. 109   Muscles of the Medial Femoral Region

iliopsoas
psoas major
pectineus
adductor longus
gracilis
adductor magnus
gluteus maximus
semimembranous
semitendinous
goose foot

anterior superior iliac spine
inguinal ligament
rectus femoris
sartorius
medial vastus
patella

Fig. 110   Position of the Patient's Leg for Therapy on the Medial Femoral Region

45°

Fig. 111   Shiatsu Points in the Medial Femoral Region

sartorius
femoral triangle
patella
adductor longus
group of adductors

Fig. 112

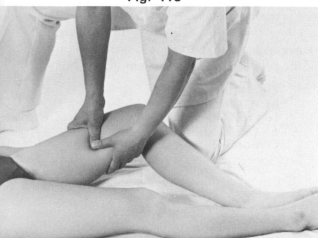

the pubic bone to a point just above the knee joint on the central part of the medial femoral region. Pressure applications last for three seconds on each point, and the therapy is repeated three times (Figs. 112 through 114).

Fig. 113

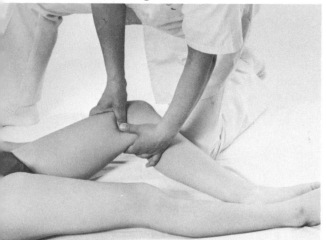

Fig. 114

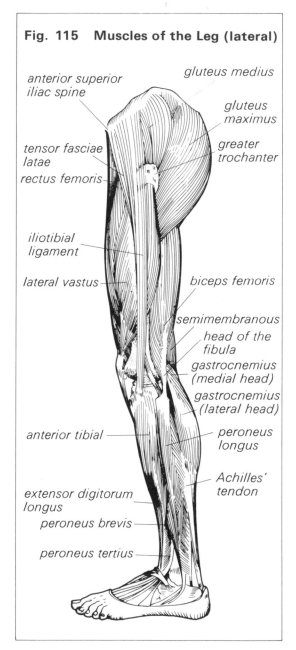

Fig. 115   Muscles of the Leg (lateral)

anterior superior iliac spine

gluteus medius

gluteus maximus

tensor fasciae latae

greater trochanter

rectus femoris

iliotibial ligament

lateral vastus

biceps femoris

semimembranous

head of the fibula

gastrocnemius (medial head)

gastrocnemius (lateral head)

anterior tibial

peroneus longus

Achilles' tendon

extensor digitorum longus

peroneus brevis

peroneus tertius

Fig. 117

Fig. 116 Shiatsu Points in the Lateral Femoral Region

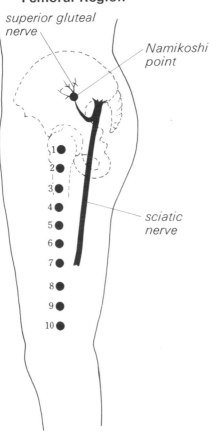

superior gluteal nerve

Namikoshi point

sciatic nerve

1 2 3 4 5 6 7 8 9 10

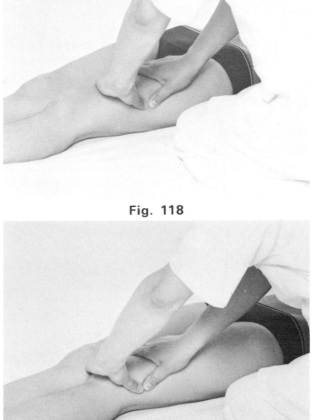

Fig. 118

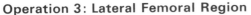

Operation 3: Lateral Femoral Region

The patient lies with both legs straight. The therapist kneels on both knees beside the patient's thigh. With both thumbs, tips just touching, the therapist applies pressure—three seconds to a point—to the ten points along the center of the lateral femoral region from the place immediately below the greater trochanter to a location immediately above the knee joint. The therapy is executed three times (Figs. 117 and 118).

Operation 4: Patellar Region

Remaining in the same posture but in a position facing the patient's knee, the therapist places thumbs and fingers in such a way as to form a frame surrounding the patella (Fig. 119). The thumbs are on the outer side of the leg, and the other fingers on the inner side. First with the left thumb, he presses for two seconds each on

Fig. 119

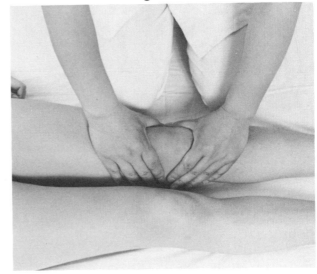

the three points moving from the outer side of the knee below the joint and inward (Fig. 120). Then with the thumb of the right hand he performs the same kind of pressure treatment on the three points that are located from the outer side of the leg inward above the knee (Fig. 120). This therapy, alterating from left to right thumbs, is repeated three times.

Fig. 120   Shiatsu Points in the Patellar Region

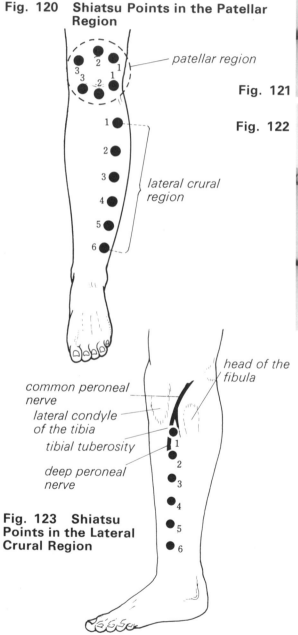

patellar region

lateral crural region

common peroneal nerve

lateral condyle of the tibia

tibial tuberosity

deep peroneal nerve

Fig. 123   Shiatsu Points in the Lateral Crural Region

head of the fibula

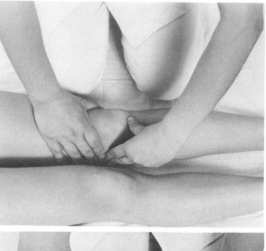

Fig. 121

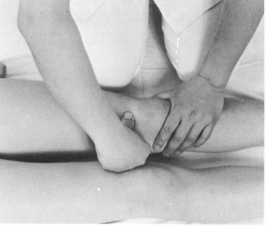

Fig. 122

Operation 5: Lateral Crural Region

Still kneeling on both knees, the therapist moves farther toward the patient's lateral crural region. The first point in the lateral crural region is about three centimenters diagonally below the tibial tuberosity and below the lateral condyle of the tibia (Fig. 123). At this point, the common peroneal nerve leaves the popliteal fossa and branches to become the superficial and deep peroneal nerves. Pressing with the thumbs causes sharp pain by forcing the deep peroneal nerve against the tibia. With thumbs overlapping, right thumb on top, and with the fingers wrapped around the inner side of the leg for support, the therapist presses the six points leading from this position down the center of the lateral crural region to the lateral malleolus (Fig. 123). Each pressure application lasts three seconds, and therapy is repeated three times (Fig. 125):

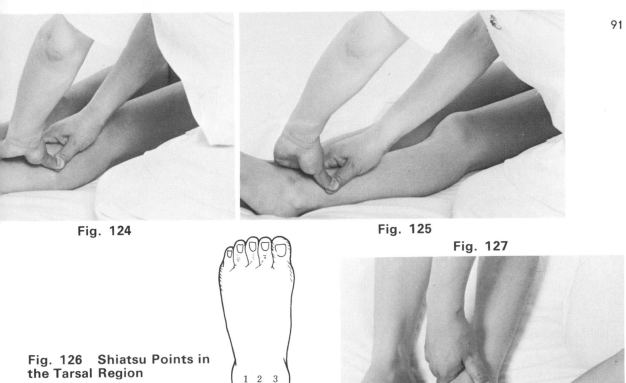

Fig. 124

Fig. 125

Fig. 127

Fig. 126 Shiatsu Points in the Tarsal Region

1 2 3

Operation 6: Tarsal Region

The therapist kneels on both knees facing the instep of the patient's left foot. Cupping the toes of the foot in his left hand to support it lightly, with the thumb of his right hand, he presses on the three points located between the lateral and medial malleoli (Fig. 126). Pressure is applied for three seconds to each point, and the therapy is repeated three times (Figs. 127 through 129).

Fig. 130 Muscles and Shiatsu Points in the Tarsal, Dorsal, and Digital Regions

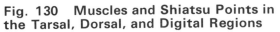

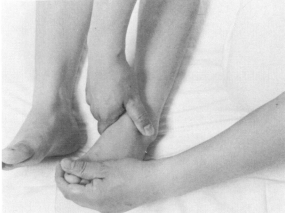

Fig. 128

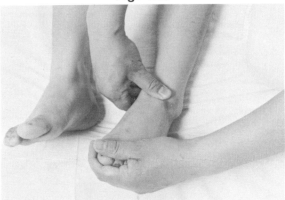

Fig. 129

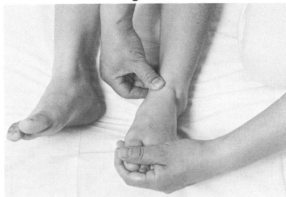

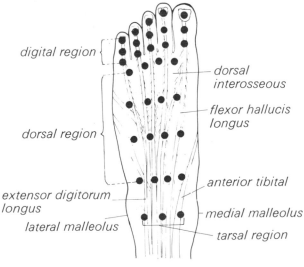

digital region

dorsal region

extensor digitorum longus

lateral malleolus

dorsal interosseous

flexor hallucis longus

anterior tibital

medial malleolus

tarsal region

Operation 7: Dorsal Region

Still cupping the patient's toes in his left hand, the therapist begins working on the instep, the pressure points on which are located on four parallel rows of four points each, beginning at the crotches of the toes and extending toward the ankle joint (Fig. 131). Starting at point 1 between the big toe and the second toe, he applies three seconds of pressure to each of the four points in this row. Then moving to the base of the second row, he continues in the same fashion until he has applied pressure once to all sixteen points (Figs. 132 and 133).

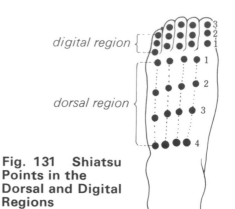

Fig. 131 Shiatsu Points in the Dorsal and Digital Regions

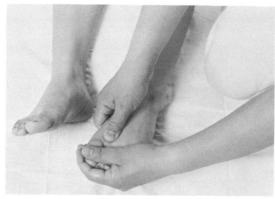

Fig. 132

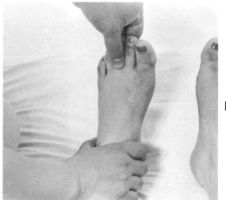

Fig. 133

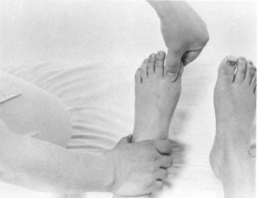

Fig. 134

Operation 8: Digital Region

Turning to kneel on both knees so that he faces the patient's ankle, the therapist cups the ankle in his right hand and applies pressure to the toe with the thumb and index finger of his left hand. The points (three to a toe) extend from the proximal to the distal phalanx. Beginning with the big toe, the therapist presses the top of each with his thumb and the underside with his index finger, two seconds for each point, until all fifteen have been treated (Figs. 134 through 136). At the conclusion of pressure on each of the third points, the toe is quickly pulled.

Fig. 135

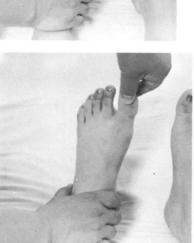

Fig. 136

Fig. 137   Ankle Exercise

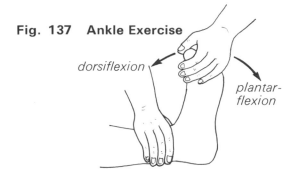

dorsiflexion

plantar-flexion

Operation 9: Toe-joint Exercise

Holding the patient's ankle with his right hand and the toes with his left hand in a wrapping fashion, the therapist performs dorsiflexion and plantarflexion of the toes (Figs. 137 through 140). The exercise must be fast and rhythmical.

Fig. 138

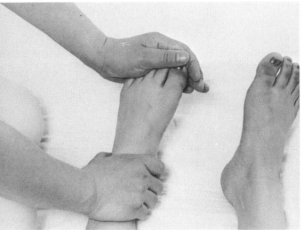

Fig. 139

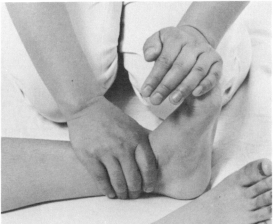

Fig. 140

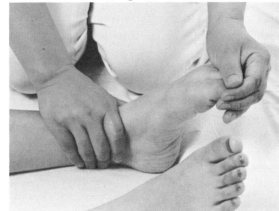

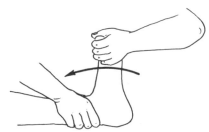

Fig. 141   Plantar Extension

Fig. 142

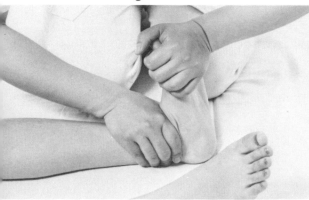

Operation 10: Plantar Extension

Placing his left hand on the ball of the sole of the foot and extending his left elbow to the side, the therapist bends the foot in the direction of the instep (Figs. 141 and 142). Once is sufficient.

Operation 11: Leg Extension

Kneeling on both knees and facing the patient's feet, with his left knee under the patient's right foot as support, the therapist uses both hands to grip the ankle joint above the heel and to lift the foot about twenty centimeters off the floor. Then, slowly leaning his body rearward, he pulls the leg for about five seconds (Figs. 143 through 145). When he has pulled it sufficiently, the therapist slowly releases it and, returning his body to its former position, lowers the patient's foot to the floor.

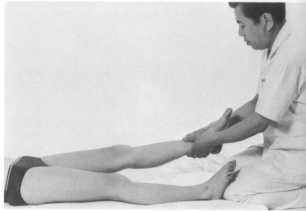

Fig. 144

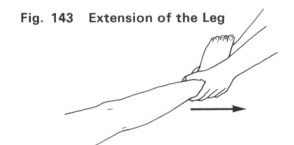

Fig. 143　Extension of the Leg

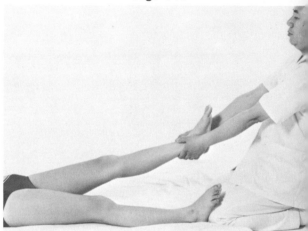

Fig. 145

Arms

Operation 1: Axillary Region

The patient extends the left arm directly to the side and turns the palm of the hand upward. The therapist kneels on both knees facing the patient's left arm in a position directed somewhat more to the axillary region than to the hand. He locates the radial artery, which passes through the wrist to the thumb, between the styloid process of the radius and the flexor pollicis longus muscle or between the flexor carpi radialis muscle and brachioradial muscle (Fig. 146). The therapist places the joined index, middle, and ring fingers of his right hand on this zone (Figs. 150 and 151). When he has found the pulse, leav-

Fig. 146　Axillary and Radial Arteries

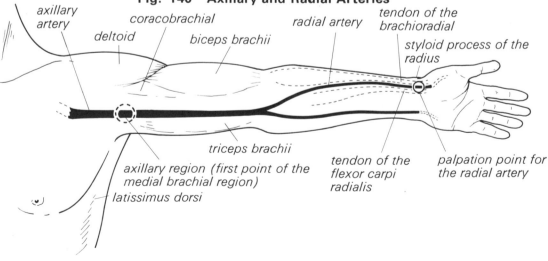

axillary artery
deltoid
coracobrachial
biceps brachii
radial artery
tendon of the brachioradial
styloid process of the radius
triceps brachii
axillary region (first point of the medial brachial region)
tendon of the flexor carpi radialis
palpation point for the radial artery
latissimus dorsi

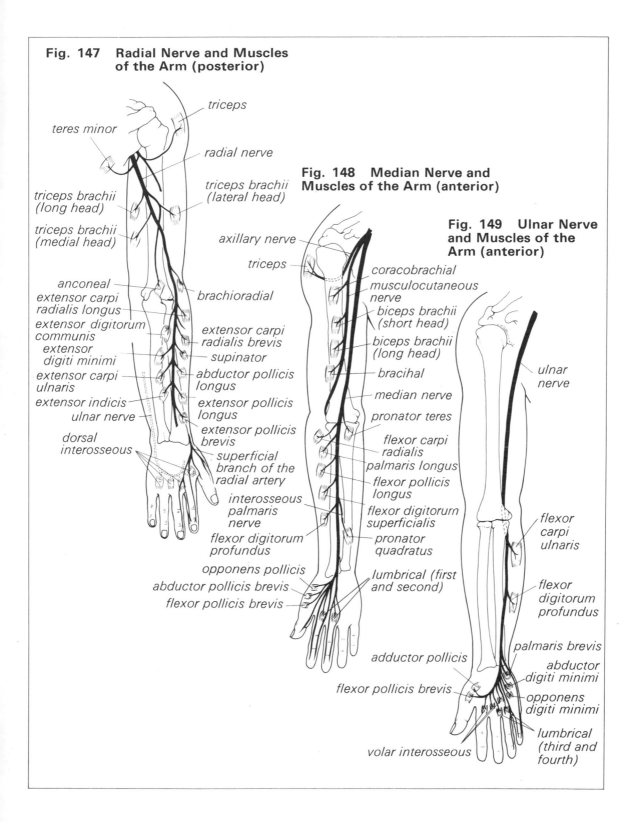

Fig. 147   Radial Nerve and Muscles of the Arm (posterior)

triceps
teres minor
radial nerve
triceps brachii (lateral head)
triceps brachii (long head)
triceps brachii (medial head)
anconeal
extensor carpi radialis longus
extensor digitorum communis
extensor digiti minimi
extensor carpi ulnaris
extensor indicis
ulnar nerve
dorsal interosseous
brachioradial
extensor carpi radialis brevis
supinator
abductor pollicis longus
extensor pollicis longus
extensor pollicis brevis
superficial branch of the radial artery
interosseous palmaris nerve
flexor digitorum profundus
opponens pollicis
abductor pollicis brevis
flexor pollicis brevis

Fig. 148   Median Nerve and Muscles of the Arm (anterior)

axillary nerve
triceps
coracobrachial
musculocutaneous nerve
biceps brachii (short head)
biceps brachii (long head)
bracihal
median nerve
pronator teres
flexor carpi radialis
palmaris longus
flexor pollicis longus
flexor digitorum superficialis
pronator quadratus
lumbrical (first and second)
adductor pollicis
flexor pollicis brevis

Fig. 149   Ulnar Nerve and Muscles of the Arm (anterior)

ulnar nerve
flexor carpi ulnaris
flexor digitorum profundus
palmaris brevis
abductor digiti minimi
opponens digiti minimi
lumbrical (third and fourth)
volar interosseous

Fig. 150 Locating the Radial Artery

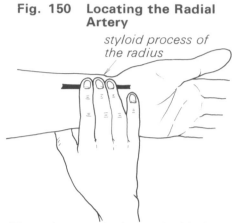

styloid process of the radius

The pulse must be located with three fingers.

Fig. 152 Locating the Axillary Artery

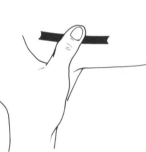

Pressing with the thumb of the left hand against the axillary artery in the armpit halts pulse in the radial artery.

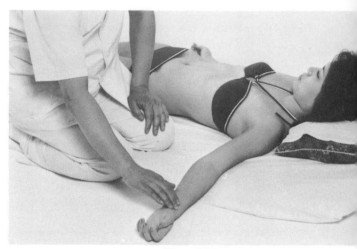

Fig. 151

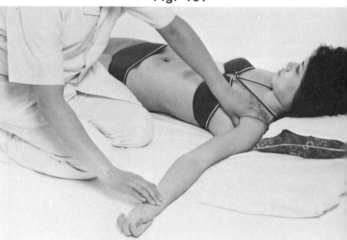

Fig. 153

Fig. 154

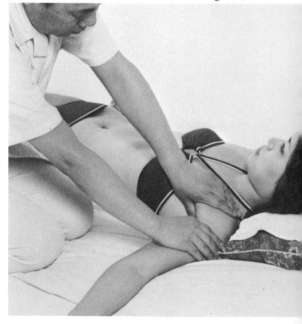

ing his right hand as it is, he presses upward (toward the suprascapular region) on the patient's axillary region with the thumb of his left hand (Figs. 152 and 153). This applies pressure to the axillary artery, passing through the axillary region, and temporarily halts pulse in the radial artery. When he can tell that this has happened, the therapist removes his right hand from the patient's arm and replaces his left thumb (on the patient's axillary region) with his right thumb and putting his left thumb on top of his right thumb, first applies firm pressure directed to the suprascapular region. Then, decreasing pressure slightly, he continues as if pulling in the direction of the elbow. Pressure lasts for five seconds on the point, and treatment is repeated three times.

Fig. 155 Shiatsu Points in the Medial Brachial Region

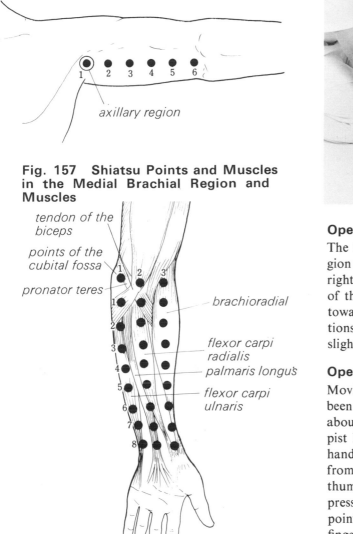

axillary region

Fig. 157 Shiatsu Points and Muscles in the Medial Brachial Region and Muscles

tendon of the biceps

points of the cubital fossa

pronator teres

brachioradial

flexor carpi radialis

palmaris longus

flexor carpi ulnaris

Fig. 156

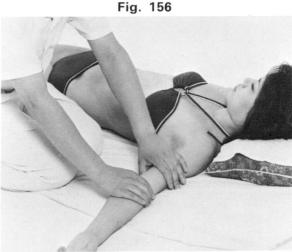

Operation 2: Medial Brachial Region

The therapist takes the point in the axillary region as point 1 and, with left thumb on top of right thumb, presses for three seconds on each of the six points (Fig. 155) leading from there toward the cubital fossa at the elbow. Applications of pressure should be made so as to pull slightly in the direction of the elbow (Fig. 156).

Operation 3: Cubital Fossa

Moving the patient's arm, which till now has been outstretched to the side, to an angle of about forty-five degrees with the body, the therapist kneels on both knees so that the patient's hand come just between them and raises his hips from the floor. With the outer edges of the thumbs barely touching each other, the therapist presses for three seconds each on the three points (Fig. 157) leading from the inner (little-finger) side to the outer (thumb) side of the patient's cubital fossa (Figs. 158 through 161).

Fig. 158

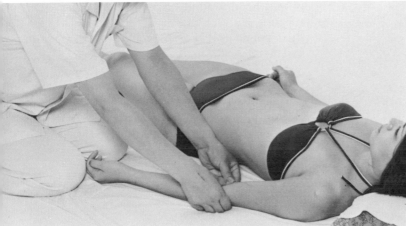

Fig. 159 Pressure Application to the Cubital Fossa

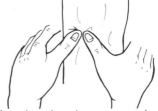

The thumbs do not overlap; their outer edges barely come into contact with each other.

Fig. 160

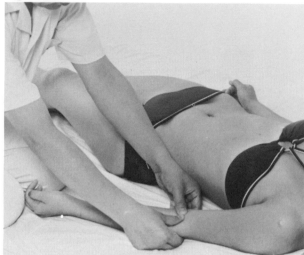

Fig. 161

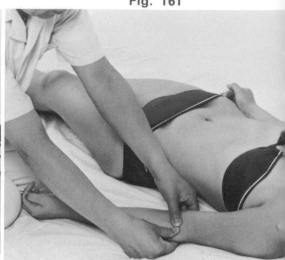

Fig. 162

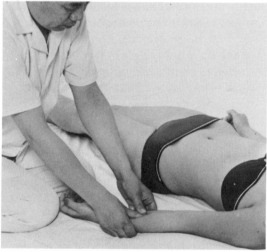

**Fig. 163 Shiatsu Points in the Delto-
pectoral Groove**

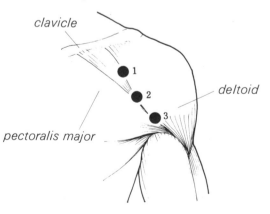

Operation 4: Medial Antebrachial Region

The therapist remains in the same position as in the preceding operation. Points for shiatsu on the medial antebrachial region are located in three parallel rows of eight points each, the first points in each row being the three points arranged horizontally just below the cubital-fossa three points (Fig. 157). With one thumb on the other, the therapist applies pressure for three seconds to each point (Fig. 162). Pressure is applied with a slight pull in the direction of the wrist.

Operation 5: Deltopectoral Groove

The patient remains in the same position, with the arm extended at forty-five degrees to the body but turns the palm down. Moving to a position facing the patient's acromion, the therapist kneels on both knees and raises his hips from the floor. Placing his right thumb on the first point on the deltopectral groove, near the clavicle (Fig. 163), he wraps the remaining fingers of that hand around the patient's shoulder for support. He then places his left thumb on his right thumb and the remaining four fingers of that hand in the patient's axillary region. The remaining points on this groove are aligned diagonally downward from the first one near the clavicle to the third one at the axillary region (Fig. 163). Pressure is applied to each one for three seconds, and therapy is repeated three times (Figs. 164 and 165).

Fig. 164 Pressure Application to the Deltopectoral Groove

The therapist kneels on both knees and raises his hips from the floor.

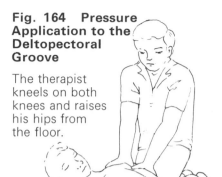

Fig. 165

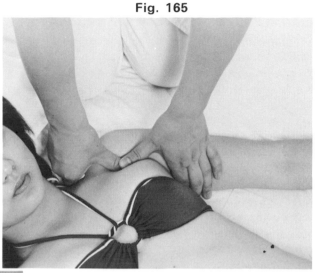

Fig. 167

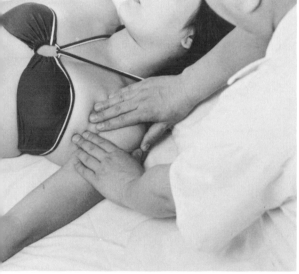

Fig. 168

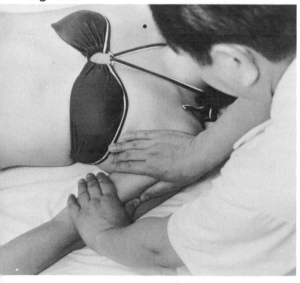

Fig. 166 Shiatsu Points in the Lateral Brachial Region

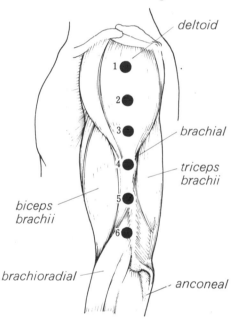

deltoid
brachial
triceps brachii
biceps brachii
brachioradial
anconeal

Operation 6: Lateral Brachial Region

The therapist kneels on both knees in front of the patient's upper arm. With the outer edges of his thumbs barely touching each other, he presses with both of them on the six points in the lateral brachial region (Fig. 166), leading from the deltoid muscle across the triceps brachii muscle and to the olecranon. Pressure is applied for three seconds on each point, and therapy is repeated three times (Figs. 167 and 168).

Operation 7: Lateral Antebrachial Region

The therapist moves to the palmar side of the patient's arm, raises her hand, and places it palm down on his own left knee. He kneels on both knees, raising his hips from the floor. The first of the eight points in the lateral antebrachial region is located on the extensor digitorum communis muscle (Fig. 169). Bending the middle finger backward causes this muscle to move in an immediately apparent way. Firm pressure on this point causes sharp pain since it forces the radial nerve against the radia. With his right thumb on the bottom, the therapist uses both thumbs to press the first point and then the remaining points leading downward from this point to the wrist. Each pressure application lasts for five seconds, and the therapy is repeated three times (Figs. 170 and 171).

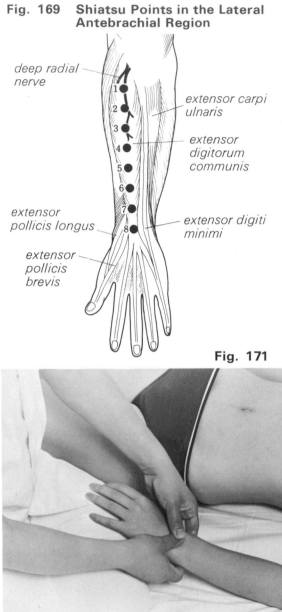

Fig. 169 Shiatsu Points in the Lateral Antebrachial Region

deep radial nerve

extensor carpi ulnaris

extensor digitorum communis

extensor pollicis longus

extensor digiti minimi

extensor pollicis brevis

Fig. 170

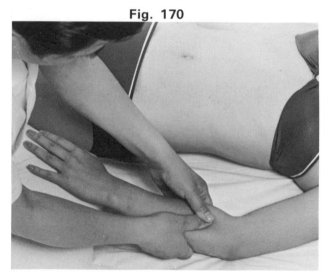

Fig. 171

Fig. 172 Shiatsu Points in the Dorsal Region

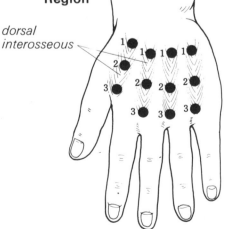

dorsal interosseous

Operation 8: Dorsal Region of the Hand

Remaining in the same posture and taking the patient's left hand in his right hand, the therapist presses with his left thumb on the rows of three points located between the proximal phalanges of the thumb and the index finger and the index finger and the middle finger (Fig. 172). Pressure lasts three seconds for each point. The remaining four fingers of the therapist's left hand are wrapped around the patient's hand for support

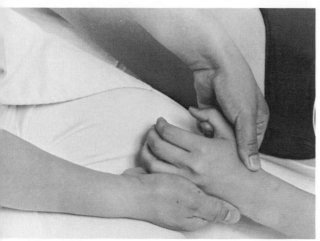

Fig. 173

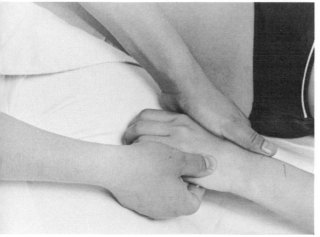

Fig. 174

**Fig. 175 Shiatsu
Points in the
Digital Region**

*right and
left sides*

palmar side

dorsal side

3

2

3

2

1

1

(Fig. 173). The therapist then takes the patient's hand in his left hand and, with his right thumb, presses on the two rows of three points between the proximal phalanges of the middle and ring fingers and the ring and little fingers. Once again pressure lasts for three seconds on each point (Fig. 174).

Operation 9: Dorsal Digital Region
Returning the patient's hand to his right hand, with the thumb and index finger of his left hand, the therapist applies pressure to the patient's thumb, index finger, and middle finger, beginning at the points at the bases of the fingers and working down the three points on the tops and bottoms of the thumbs and four points on the tops and bottoms of the other two fingers and then on the points on the right and left sides of the fingers (Fig. 175). The patient's fingers are held between the therapist's thumb and index finger, and pressure is applied for two seconds to a point. Each finger is pulled at the conclusion of pressure application on the last point (Figs. 176 through 178). When the middle finger has been treated, the therapist shifts the patient's hand into his own right hand and treats the remaining fingers with his left thumb and index finger.

Fig. 176

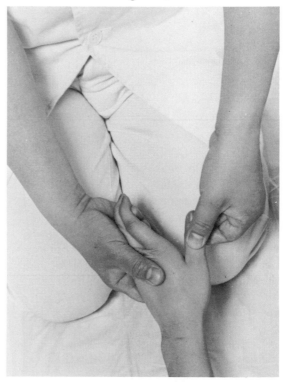

Fig. 177

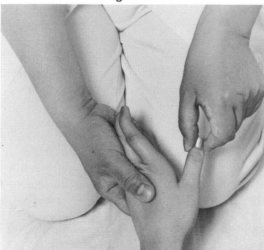

Fig. 178

Fig. 179

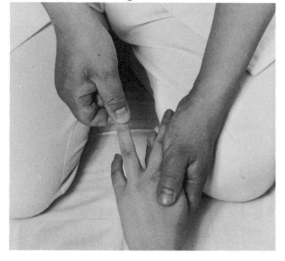

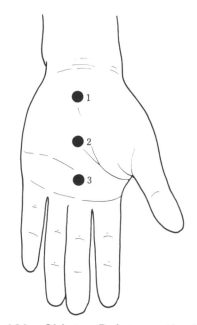

Fig. 180   Shiatsu Points on the Palm

Operation 10: Palm

Remaining in the same position, the therapist turns the patient's hand palm up. Bringing the outer edges of his thumbs together on the palm, he wraps the remaining fingers of both hands around the patient's hand for support. The points for pressure application (Fig. 180) are located on the carpus, or base of the hand, in the center of the palm, and at the base of the middle finger. With both thumbs—outer edges barely touching each other—the therapist applies pressure for three seconds to each point and repeats this therapy three times (Figs. 181 through 183). Then to the second point—center of the palm—with the left thumb on the right thumb, he applies strong pressure with both for five seconds. Treatment is repeated three times (Fig. 184). Leaning his trunk rearward, he pulls the patient's arm (Figs. 185 and 186).

Fig. 181

Fig. 182

Fig. 183

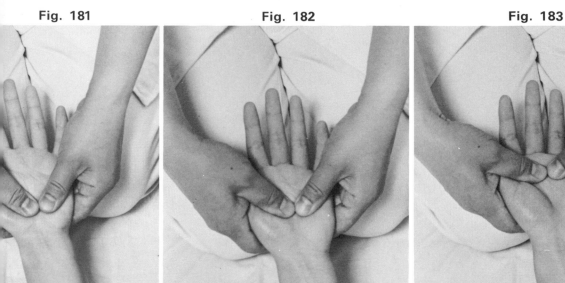

Fig. 184

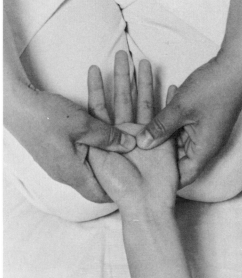

With overlapping thumbs still pressed against the patient's thumb, the therapist leans his trunk rearward to extend the patient's arm.

Fig. 185   Extension of the Arm

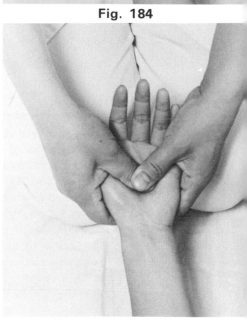

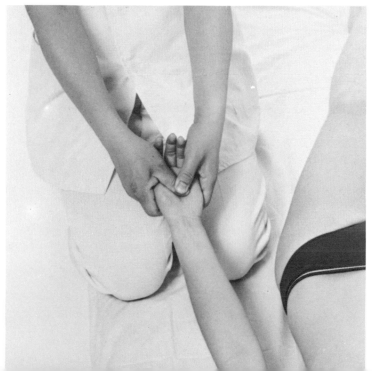

Fig. 186

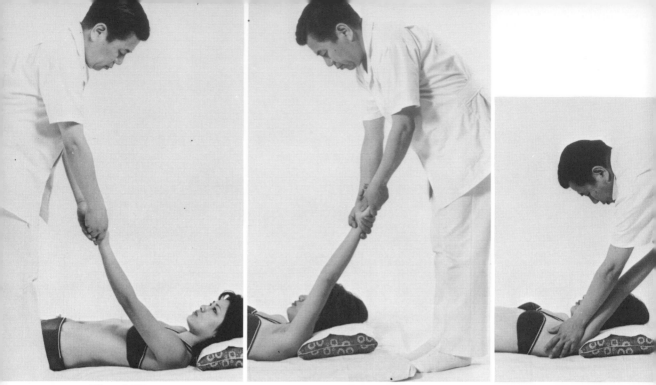

Fig. 187   Fig. 188   Fig. 189

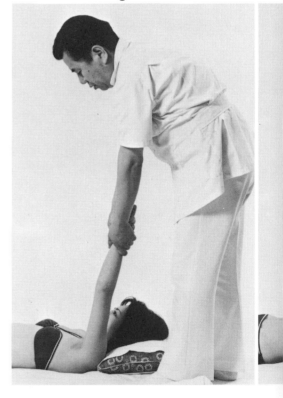

Fig. 192

Operation 11: Extension of the Arm

Still holding the patient's hand at the end of the preceding operation, the therapist stands and walks behind her head to a position above her left shoulder (Figs. 187 and 188). Gripping the arm at the wrist and keeping it well extended, he lowers it until it forms an angle of forty-five degrees with the floor. Holding the patient's wrist in his right hand, with his left hand, the therapist strokes the upper arm from the armpit three times (Figs. 189 and 190). Gripping the wrist with both hands again, he lowers the arm, still extended, slowly to the floor. When, it is fully lowered, the arm should form an angle of 180 degrees with the body and should lie close beside the ear (Fig. 191). Relaxing it, the therapist slowly raises the arm to the vertical position then lightly pulls it once. Next, relaxing it again, he allows it to fall lightly forward (Figs. 192 through 195).

This completes therapy for a patient in a supine position on the left leg and arm. The same therapy is repeated on the right leg and arm.

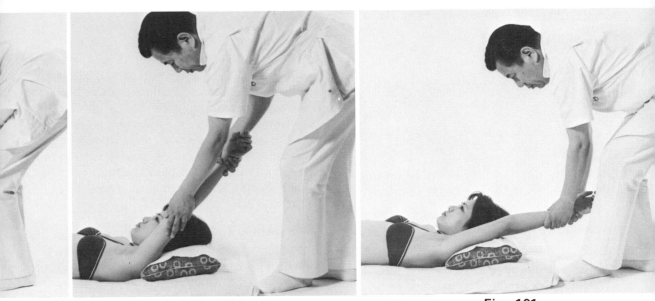

Fig. 190   Fig. 191

Fig. 193   Fig. 194   Fig. 195

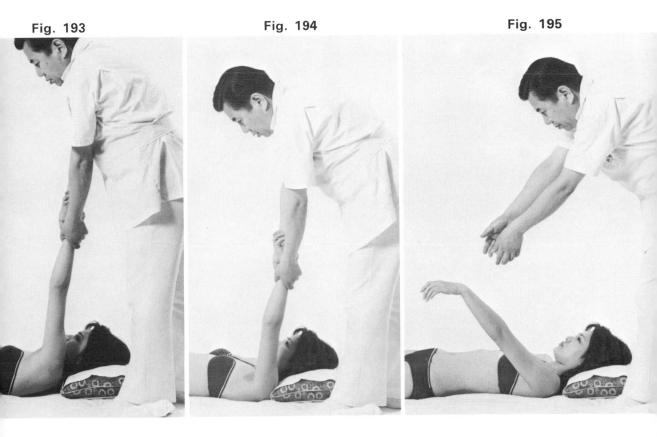

106

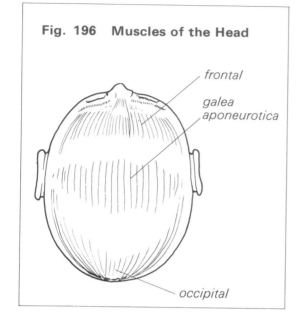

Fig. 196   Muscles of the Head

frontal

galea
aponeurotica

occipital

Fig. 197   Six Points on the
Median Line

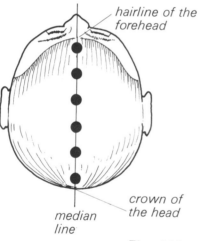

hairline of the
forehead

crown of
the head

median
line

Head

Operation 1: Median Line

The therapist moves to a position at the crown of the patient's head and kneels on both knees. It is a good idea to place a thin towel or other suitable cloth on the patient's head for this therapy. With both thumbs—right thumb on the bottom —the therapist presses for three seconds on each of the six points (Fig. 196) leading from the hairline to the crown of the head on the median line. The therapy is repeated three times (Figs. 198 through 200).

Operation 2: Temporal Region

The therapist puts his right palm lightly on the patient's right temporal region for support. Shiatsu points (Fig. 201) for the left temporal region are arranged in six rows leading to the left from the six points on the median line. The

Fig. 198

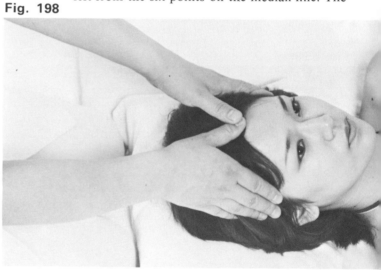

Fig. 199

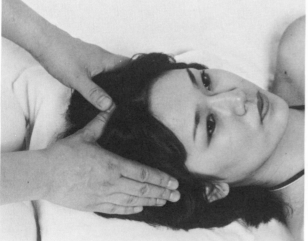

Fig. 200

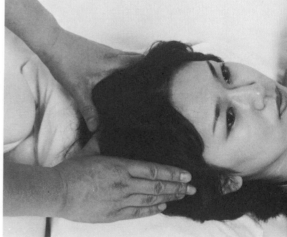

Fig. 201 Shiatsu Points in the Temporal Region

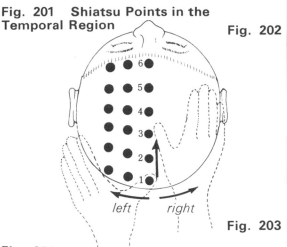

left   right

Fig. 202

Fig. 203

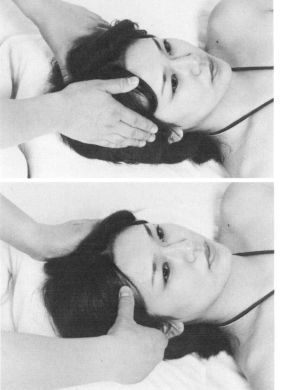

Fig. 204

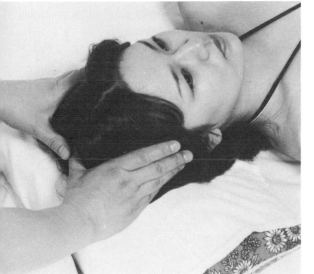

Fig. 205

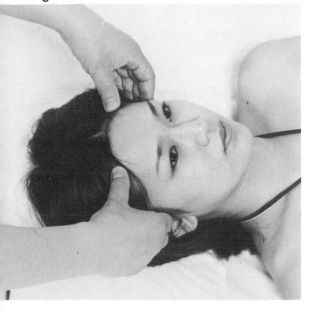

first point for treatment on the temporal region is the final point on the median line. Using his left thumb, the therapist presses each of the points in each row for three seconds (Fig. 202). Then, placing his left palm on the patient's left temporal region for support, he performs the same therapy on the corresponding six rows of points in the right temporal region.

Operation 3: Median Line and Temporal Region

First with overlapping thumbs—right thumb on the bottom—the therapist presses once on each of the points on the median line, beginning with the hairline on the forehead and moving toward the crown of the head. Then, with thumbs, the outer edges of which touch each other, starting at the last point at the crown of the head on the median line, he simultaneously presses each point in the temporal right and left rows. Moving toward the hairline on the forehead, he continues until he has pressed all points once for two seconds each. Then, with overlapping thumbs, he returns to the first median-line point, at the hairline on the forehead, and presses each with both thumbs, ending with a five-second pressure application on the final point on the crown of the head on the median line.

Face

Operation 1: Frontal and Nasal Regions

Remaining in the same position but raising his hips from the floor, the therapist presses three seconds on each of the three frontal points (Fig. 206) along the facial median line from the glabella, between the eyebrows, to the forehead hairline with both thumbs—right thumb on the bottom. The therapy is repeated three times (Figs. 209 through 211). Lowering his hips, with the overlapped index and middle fingers of each hand—index finger on top—he presses simultaneously on each of the nasal points in the rows leading from the root of the nose to the wings of the nostrils. Each pressure application lasts for three seconds. One application for each point is sufficient (Figs. 212 through 214). In this treat-

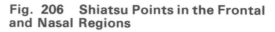

Fig. 206   Shiatsu Points in the Frontal and Nasal Regions

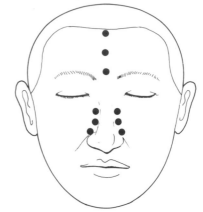

ment, the therapist must be careful not to press directly on the wings of the nostrils in such a way as to close the nasal passage.

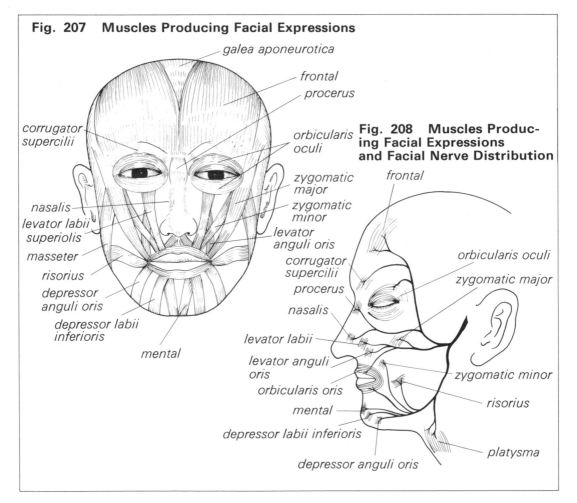

Fig. 207   Muscles Producing Facial Expressions

galea aponeurotica
frontal
procerus
corrugator supercilii
orbicularis oculi
zygomatic major
zygomatic minor
nasalis
levator labii superiolis
levator anguli oris
masseter
risorius
depressor anguli oris
depressor labii inferioris
mental

Fig. 208   Muscles Producing Facial Expressions and Facial Nerve Distribution

frontal
orbicularis oculi
zygomatic major
corrugator supercilii
procerus
nasalis
levator labii
levator anguli oris
orbicularis oris
mental
depressor labii inferioris
depressor anguli oris
zygomatic minor
risorius
platysma

Fig. 209

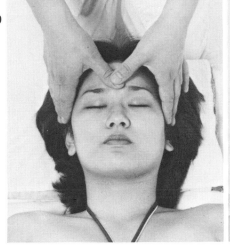

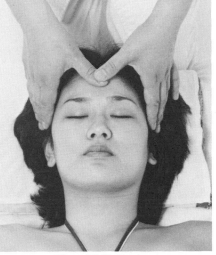

Fig. 210 ▲

Fig. 211
▶

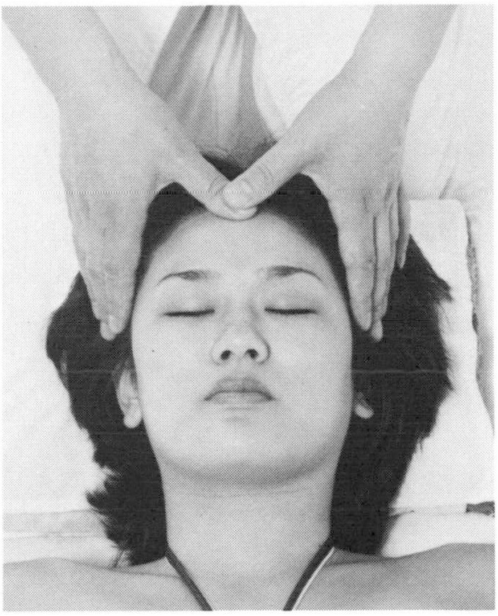

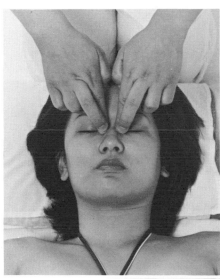

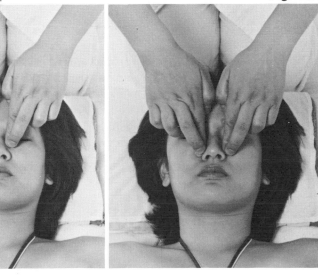

Fig. 212 ▲

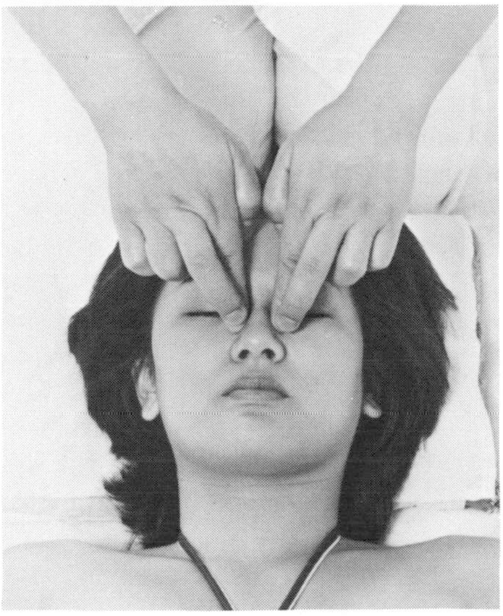

Fig. 214

Fig. 213
▶

Fig. 215   Fig. 216   Fig. 217

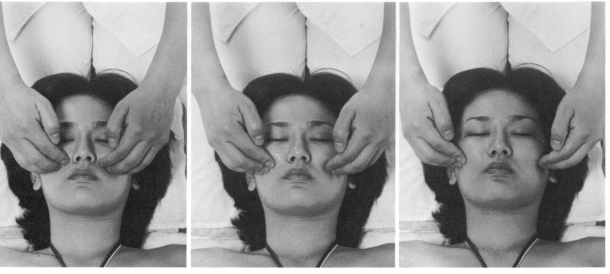

Fig. 218   Shiatsu Points in the Zygomatic and Orbital Regions

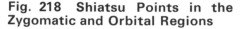

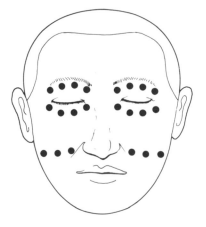

Fig. 219

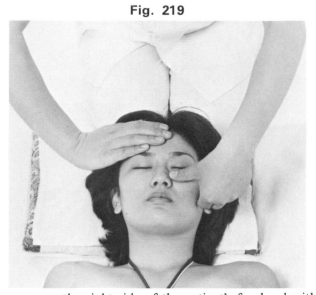

Operation 2: Zygomatic, Orbital, and Temple Regions

In the same position, with the index, middle, and ring fingers of each hand, the therapist presses on the two rows of three points leading to the side from the nose along the lower border of the zygomatic bone (Fig. 218) simultaneously for three seconds on each point. The therapy is executed only once. The therapist applies pressure with a light pull toward himself (Figs. 215 through 217).

To treat the orbital region and temples, the therapist rests the palm of his right hand lightly on the right side of the patient's forehead with fingers turned inward. Then, with the thumb of his left hand, he presses each of the four points (Figs. 219 through 222) in the infraorbital region from the inside corner to the outside corner of the eye for three seconds each. The therapy is performed only once. Then he presses on each of the four points in the supraorbital region with the thumb of his left hand in the same way (Figs. 223 and 224). Then, with the thumb of the left hand, he presses the three points leading from the outer corner of the right eye across the right temple in the direction of the ear (Fig. 225). Pres-

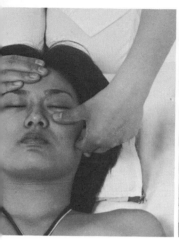

Fig. 220

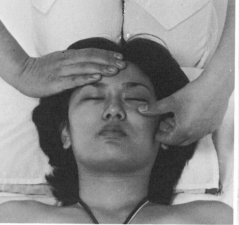

Fig. 221

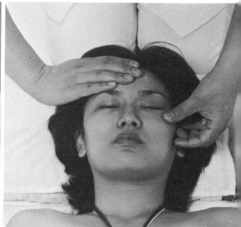

Fig. 222

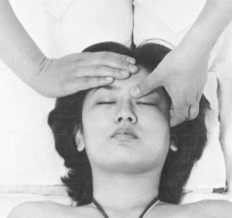

Fig. 223

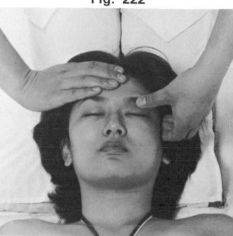

Fig. 224

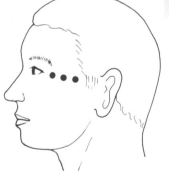

Fig. 225 Shiatsu Points on the Temples

sure is applied for three seconds on each point, and therapy is performed only once. When treatment is completed on the left orbital and temple regions, the hands are changed; and therapy is performed in the same way on the right orbital and temple regions.

Fig. 226

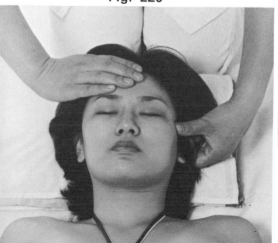

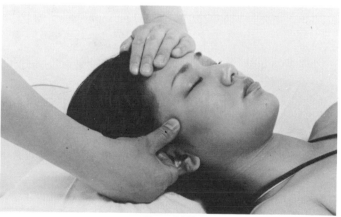

Fig. 227

Operation 3: Palm Pressure on the Eyeballs

With the fingers of both hands brought tips together in the center of the patient's face, the therapist lightly places the palms of both hands over the eyeballs and applies simultaneous pressure to both for ten seconds (Fig. 228). Before performing this treatment, the therapist should cover the patient's eyes with a clean towel or other suitable cloth.

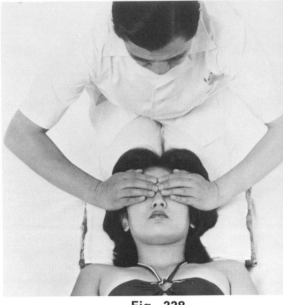

Fig. 228

Chest

Operation 1: Intercostal Region

Remaining in the same position in which he performed therapy on the face, the therapist rests his right hand—thumb spread—on the patient's chest near the shoulder for support. With the thumb of the left hand, he treats the intercostal muscles (internal and external). Points for such treatment are located between the ribs in six rows beginning at the sternal body and moving outward to the sides (Fig. 229). Pressure is applied with the left thumb for two seconds on each point; and therapy is performed only once (Figs. 230 through 232). Next, placing the left hand on the patient's upper chest for support and using the thumb of the right hand, the therapist performs the same therapy on the right intercostal muscles.

Fig. 229 Shiatsu Points in the Pectoral Region

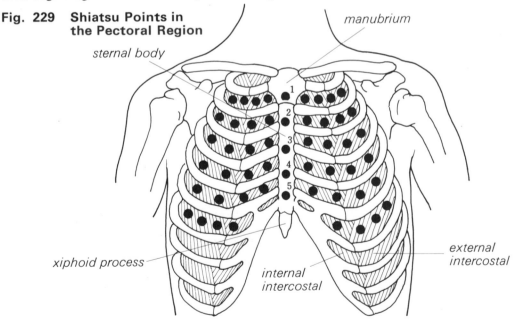

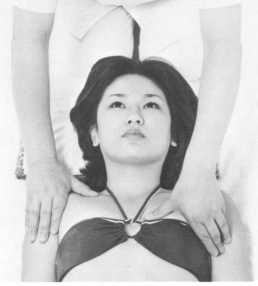

Fig. 230

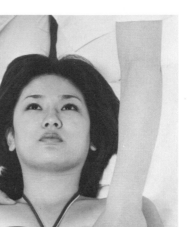

Fig. 231

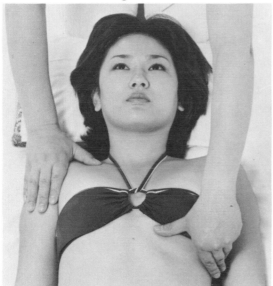

Fig. 232

Operation 2: Circular Palm Pressure on the Sternal and Pectoral Regions

In the same position, using both thumbs with the tips brought together, the therapist applies pressure for three seconds on each of the five points leading from just below the manubrium forward to the xiphoid process (Fig. 229). Therapy is repeated three times (Figs. 233 and 234). Pressure must be neither strong nor sudden and must not be applied directly to the xiphoid process.

Fig. 234

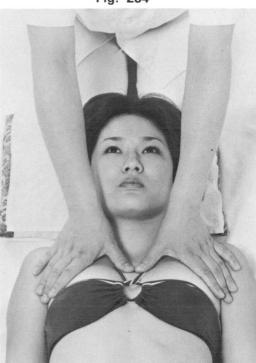

Fig. 233 Treatment for the Sternal Body

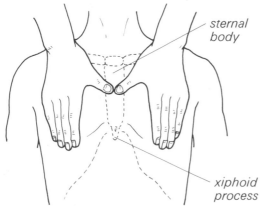

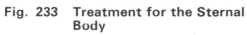

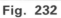

sternal body

xiphoid process

Fig. 235 Circular Pressure on the Pectoral Region

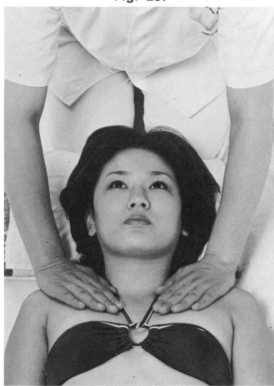

The therapist applies circular rotational pressure in the direction of the arrow.

Next, simultaneously with the palms of both hands, the therapist performs rotational pressure (ten times) on the patient's pectoral region (chest) in the outward direction (Fig. 235). Finally, returning both palms to the upper pectoral region and holding them well against the patient's body, the therapist strokes downward across the pectoral region simultaneously and has the patient exhale as he does so (Figs. 236 through 238). This therapy is performed twice. Then the palms are returned to the patient's upper pectoral region and released.

Fig. 236 Downward Pressure on the Pectoral Region

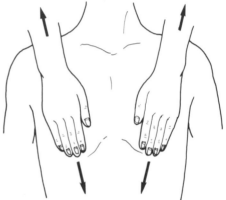

Fig. 237

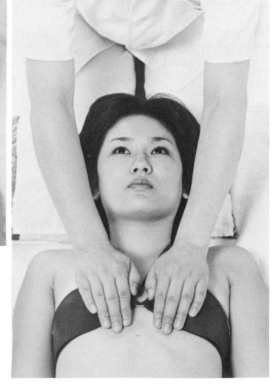

Fig. 238

Abdomen

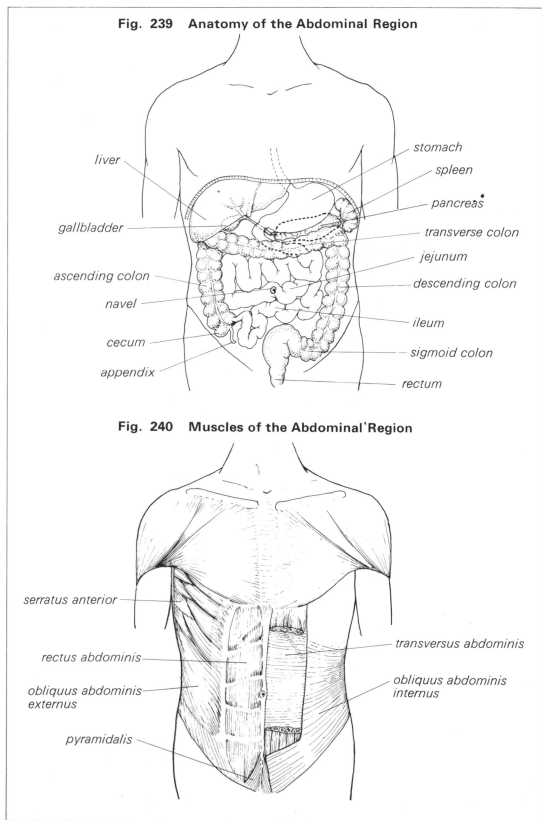

Fig. 239   Anatomy of the Abdominal Region

liver
gallbladder
ascending colon
navel
cecum
appendix

stomach
spleen
pancreas
transverse colon
jejunum
descending colon
ileum
sigmoid colon
rectum

Fig. 240   Muscles of the Abdominal Region

serratus anterior
rectus abdominis
obliquus abdominis externus
pyramidalis

transversus abdominis
obliquus abdominis internus

116

Operation 1: Palm Pressure Series

The therapist kneels on both knees facing the patient's right lateral abdominal region. Remaining prone, the patient either places both hands on the chest or extends the right arm outward to the right side and the left arm along the left side of the body. Putting his left palm flat on his own left knee, with the right palm, the therapist investigates and presses the following points in the order given: 1. upper stomach or epigastric fossa, 2. small intestine, 3. bladder, 4. cecum, 5. liver, 6. spleen, 7. descending colon, 8. sigmoid colon, and 9. rectum (Figs. 239 and 241). Each application lasts for three seconds, and the therapy is repeated three times (Figs. 242 through 250).

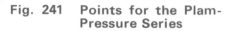

Fig. 241 Points for the Plam-Pressure Series

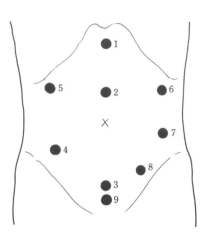

Fig. 242

Fig. 243

Fig. 244

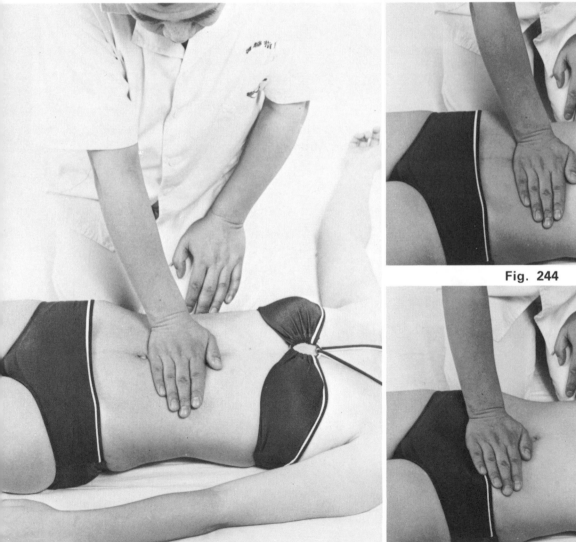

117

Fig. 245

Fig. 246

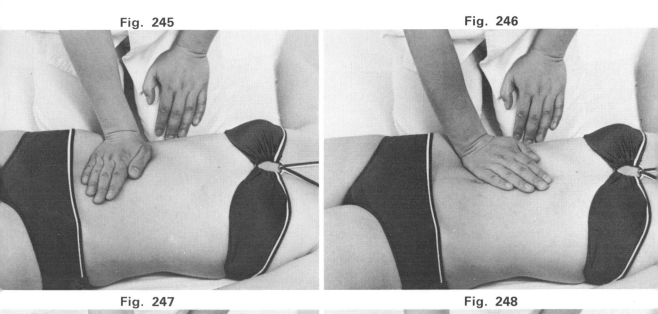

Fig. 247

Fig. 248

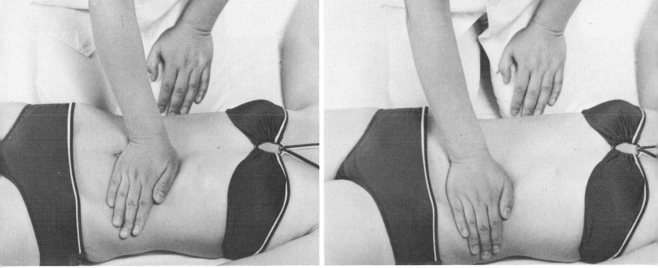

Fig. 249

Fig. 250

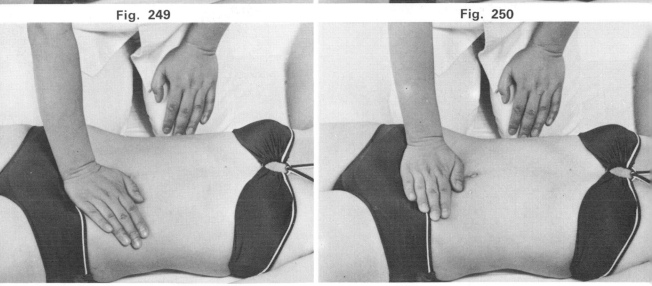

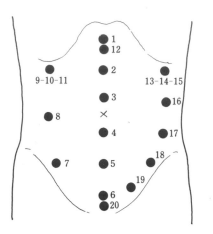

Fig. 251   Twenty Points on the Abdomen

Operation 2: Twenty Points on the Abdomen

The therapist kneels on his right knee, near the patient's right buttock. His left knee and hips are raised. The twenty abdominal points (Fig. 251) are 1, 2, and 3 from the epigastric fossa to just above the navel; 4, 5, and 6 from immediately below the navel to the bladder; 7 at the location of the cecum; 8 at the ascending colon; and 9, 10, and 11 at the liver; 12 at the stomach; 13, 14, and 15 at the gallbladder; 16, 17, and 18 at the descending colon; 19 at the sigmoid colon; and 20 at the rectum. The outer edges of the thumbs are brought together, and the other fingers are spread to the sides to form a W with the thumbs. Pressure is applied in synchronization with the patient's breathing. Each pressure application lasts three seconds, and all twenty points are treated three times (Figs. 252 through 268).

Fig. 252

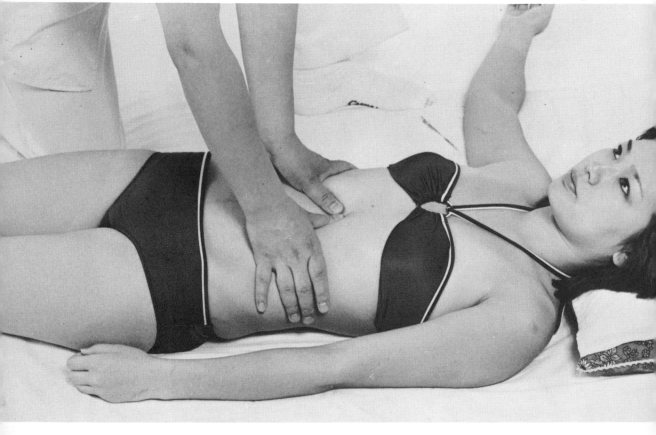

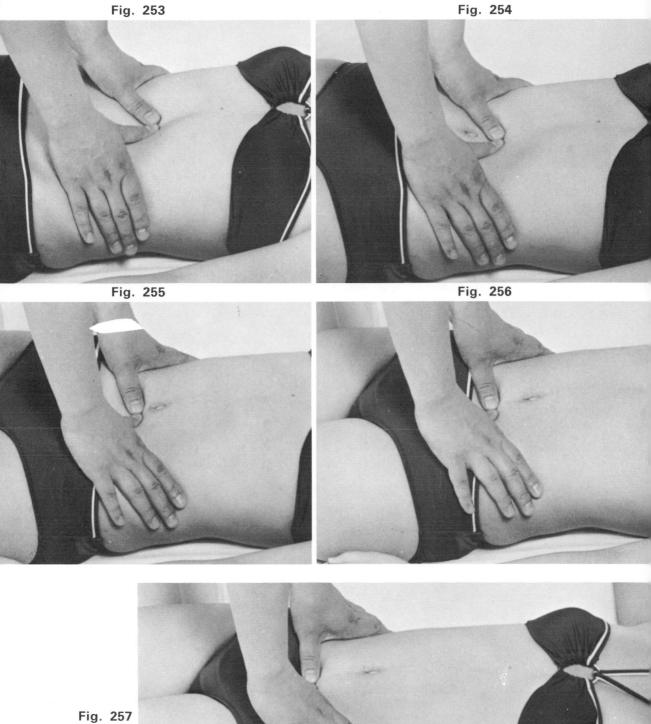

Fig. 253

Fig. 254

Fig. 255

Fig. 256

Fig. 257

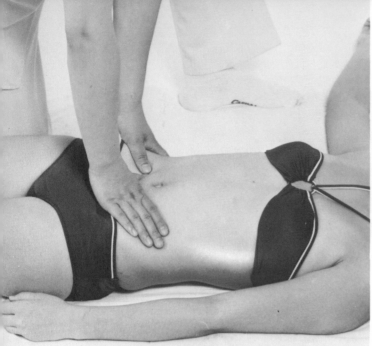

Fig. 258

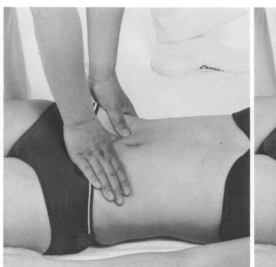

Fig. 259

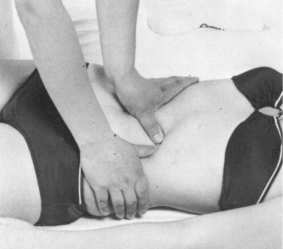

Fig. 263

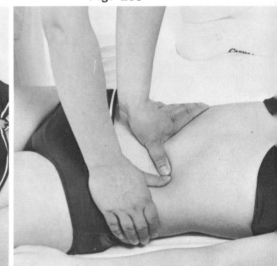

Fig. 264

Fig. 266

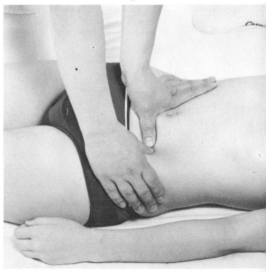

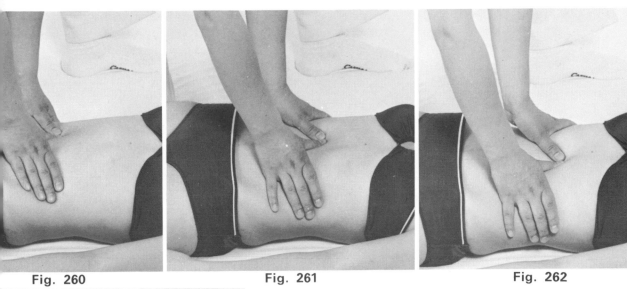

Fig. 260   Fig. 261   Fig. 262

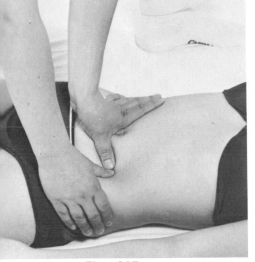

Fig. 268

Fig. 265

Fig. 267

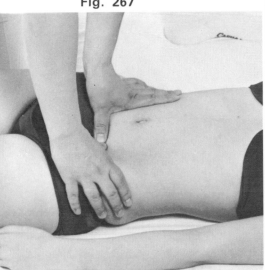

Fig. 269 Shiatsu Points in the Small-intestine Region

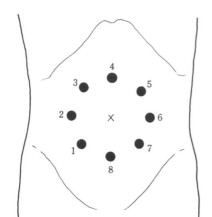

Operation 3: Small-intestine Region

Remaining in the same position, with both thumbs held so that their outer edges touch each other, the therapist applies three seconds of pressure on each of the eight points at the small intestine (Fig. 269). The pressure applications start from a place diagonally to the right (patient's right) and above the navel and are treated in clockwise, circular order. Therapy is repeated three times.

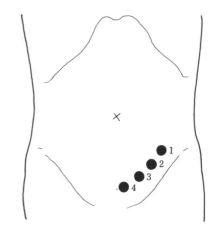

Fig. 270 Shiatsu Points in the Region of the Sigmoid Colon

Operation 4: Region of the Sigmoid Colon

Remaining in the same position as for the preceding operation, the therapist rests his left palm lightly on the patient's anterior superior iliac spine for support. With the digital ball of his right thumb, moving in small stages from point 1, he presses for three seconds on each of the four points for the sigmoid colon (Fig. 270). Therapy is repeated three times (Fig. 271).

Fig. 271

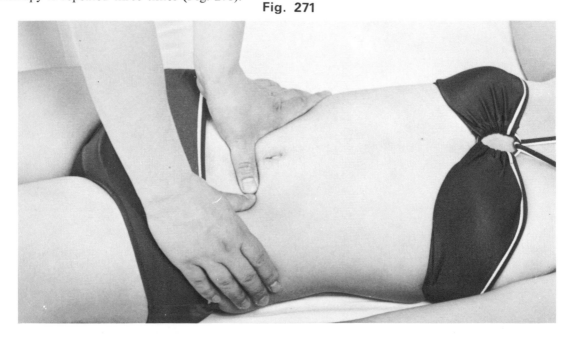

Fig. 272   Rippling Palm Pressure and Circular Palm Pressure

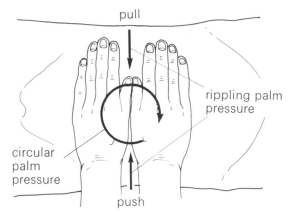

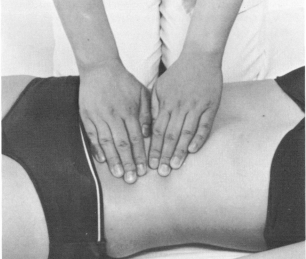

Fig. 273

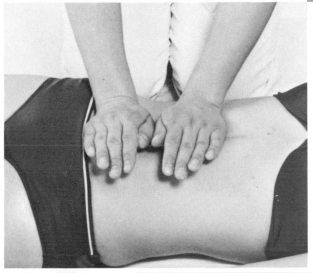

Fig. 274 ▲

Operation 5: Rippling Palm Pressure

Returning to a kneeling position, on both knees, facing the patient's abdomen, the therapist places both palms together on the patient's left lateral abdominal region, fingers pointed straight forward and hand centered on the navel. Simultaneously, with the four fingers of both hands, he pulls the area of the sigmoid colon and pushes the area of the ascending colon with the carpi of both hands (Figs. 272 through 275). He repeats this rippling pulling and pushing action five times.

Fig. 275
▶

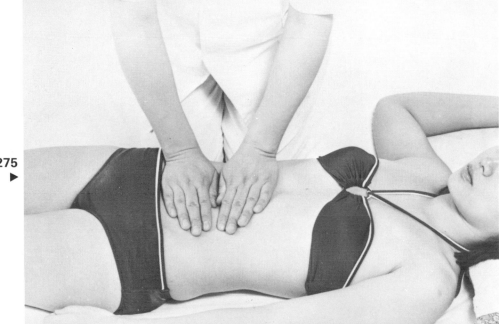

124

Operation 6: Circular Palm Pressure and Vibrational Palm Pressure

Raising his hips, though otherwise remaining in the same position as in the preceding operation, the therapist places both palms on the center of the patient's abdomen. Pressing his hands firmly against the patient's body in a way that exerts mild, penetrating suction, he exerts circular palm pressure in the clockwise direction ten times (Fig. 272). He then administers ten seconds of vibrational pressure with both palms (Fig. 276).

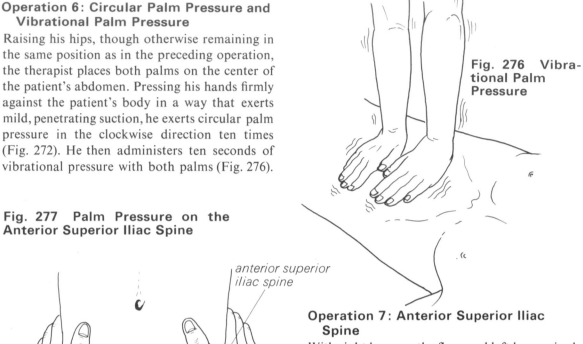

Fig. 276 Vibrational Palm Pressure

Fig. 277 Palm Pressure on the Anterior Superior Iliac Spine

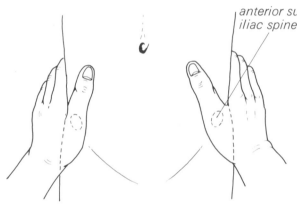

anterior superior iliac spine

Operation 7: Anterior Superior Iliac Spine

With right knee on the floor and left knee raised, the therapist kneels at the right side of the patient's right thigh and raises his hips. With the digital balls of his thumbs on the patient's right and left anterior superior iliac spine, alternately with the left then the right palm, he applies vertically directed pressure (Figs. 227 through 229). Application on one side lasts for one second, and the series is repeated rhythmically ten times.

Fig. 278   Fig. 279

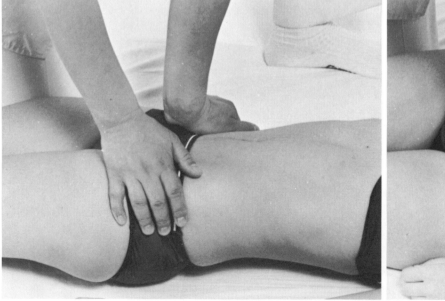

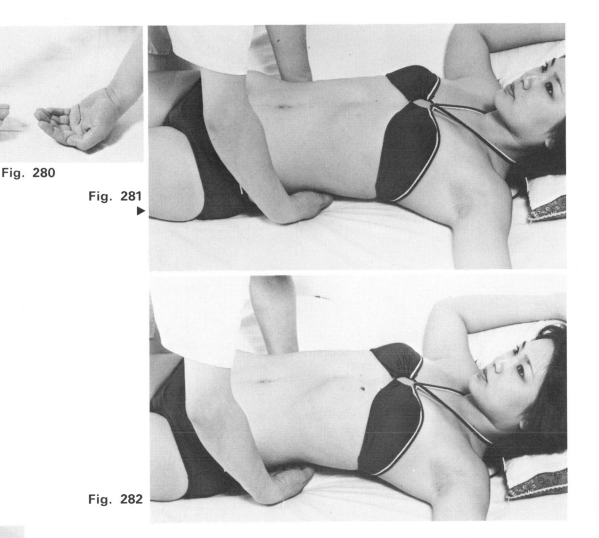

Fig. 280

Fig. 281 ▶

Fig. 282

Operation 8: Upward-kneading of the Abdominal Region

Remaining in the same position and holding the fingers of both hands together with palms upward (Fig. 280), the therapist slides both hands under the patient's body until the tips of his fingers reach points directly below the navel and to the sides of the third lumbar vertebra. Then, using the digital balls of the fingers, he applies an upward kneading motion (Figs. 281 and 282). During this operation, the backs of the hands remain on the floor and do not move. The four fingers should make use of the lever principle. The therapy is repeated three times. To avoid interfering with the therapist's work, the patient must bend both arms upward at the elbows.

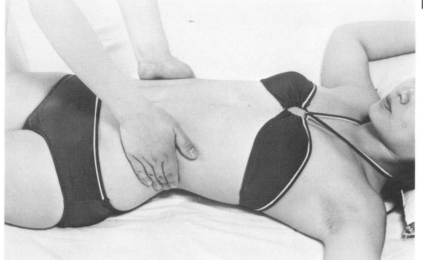

Fig. 283

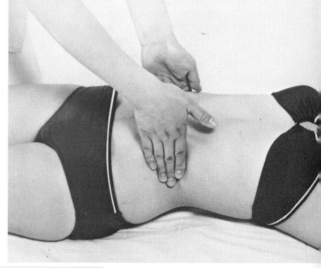

Fig. 284

Operation 9: Lateral Abdominal Region

Remaining in the same posture, the therapist places his palms on both lateral abdominal regions of the patient's body. The four fingers of each hand are held together, and their tips are pointed downward. He pulls his hands simultaneously upward, pressing both lateral abdominal regions (Figs. 283 through 285). This is repeated three times at fast speed. When the hands are raised from the patient's abdomen, the palms must face each other.

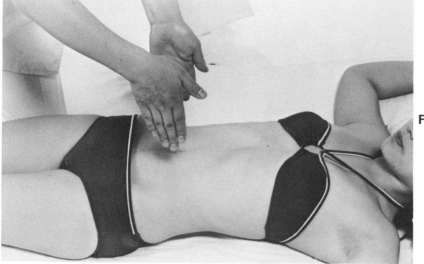

Fig. 285

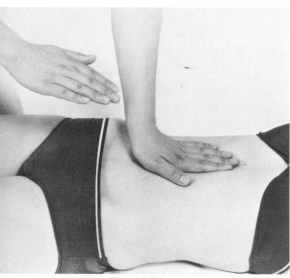

Operation 10: Palm Pressure and Vibrational Pressure on the Abdominal Region

Remaining in the same position, the therapist strokes the patient's abdomen from the epigastric fossa downward rapidly and smoothly ten times, alternating with first the left and then the right palm (Figs. 286 through 288). Then he places his right palm—fingers pointed toward the epigastric fossa—over the patient's navel, puts his left palm on his right hand, at ninety-degree angles, and applies ten seconds of vibrational pressure (Fig. 289).

Fig. 286

Fig. 287 ▶

Fig. 288

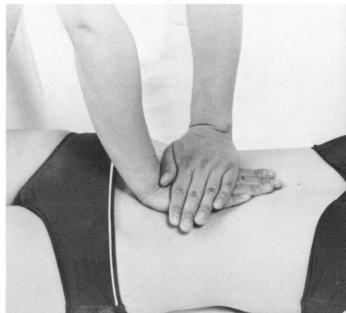

Fig. 289

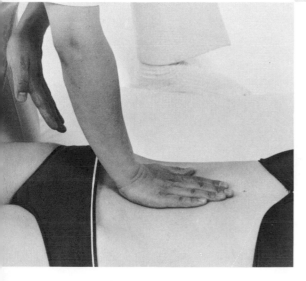

128

Total-body Treatment Using a Therapy Table

A table for shiatsu treatment should come to about the height of the tops of the therapist's knees and should be from 60 to 70 centimeters wide and from 180 to 190 centimeters long. It must be firm and without springs; an ordinary bed spoils treatment by bouncing.

Advantages of the Therapy Table

1. Since with a table he works standing, the therapist can apply pressure more easily and can move from part to part of the patient's body more rapidly.
2. Even patients suffering from paralysis, hernia of the intervertebral discs, or ailments of the joints can more easily assume therapy postures on a table.
3. As shall be discussed later, it is difficult to treat the legs of people with damage in this part of the body. The use of a table makes it possible for such patients to sit on the edge in postures permitting effective treatment.

Shiatsu for a Patient Lying in the Lateral Position

Fig. 1 Anterior Cervical Region   **Fig. 2 Lateral Cervical Region**

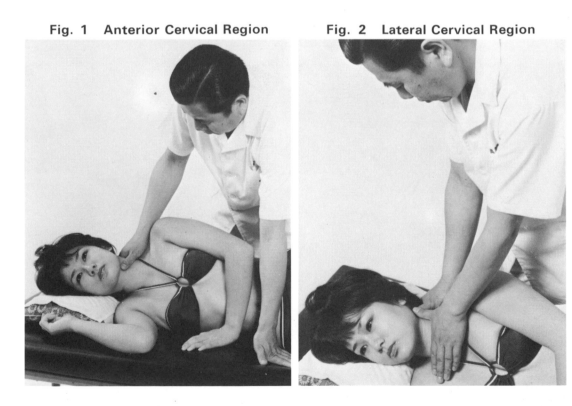

Fig. 3   Medulla Oblongata

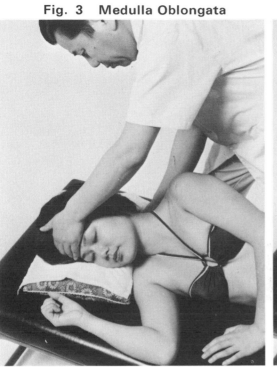

Fig. 4   Posterior Cervical Region

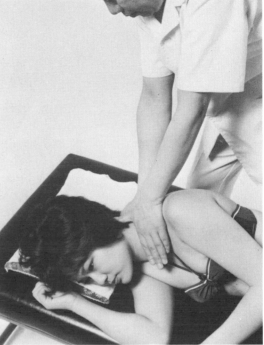

Fig. 5   Suprascapular Region

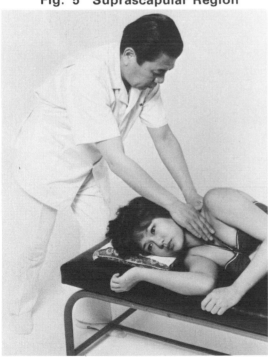

Fig. 6   Interscapular Region

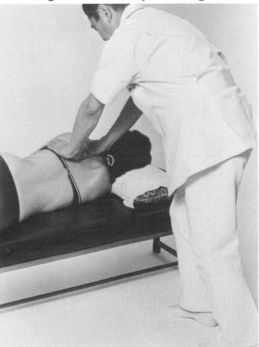

130

Fig. 7 Infrascapular and Lumbar Regions

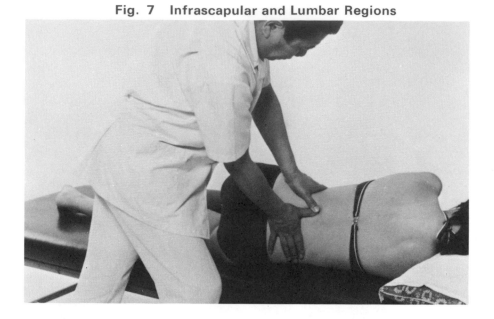

Shiatsu for a Patient Lying in the Prone Position

Fig. 8 Occipital Region

Fig. 9 Medulla Oblongata

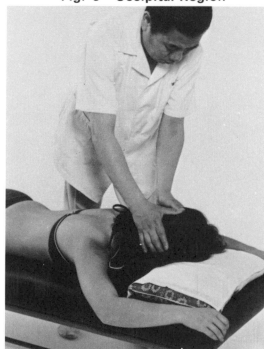
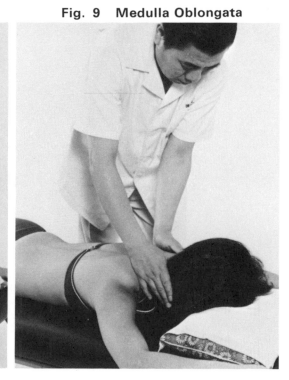

Fig. 10 Posterior Cervical Region

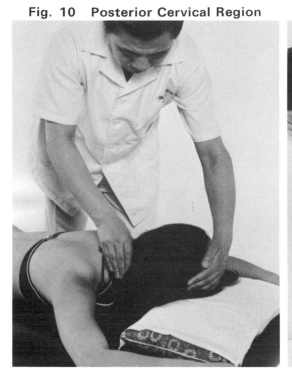

Fig. 11 Suprascapular Region

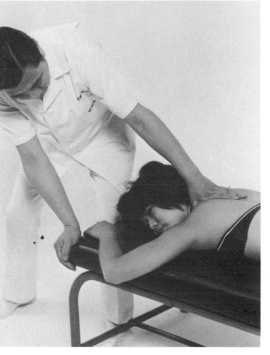

Fig. 12 Interscapular Region

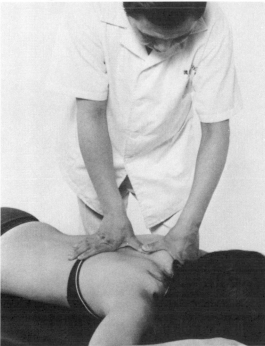

Fig. 13 Lumbar Region

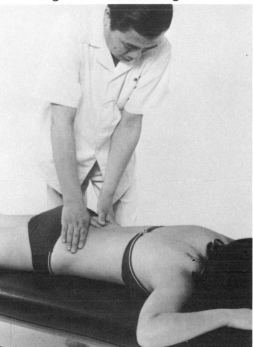

132

Fig. 14　Namikoshi Point

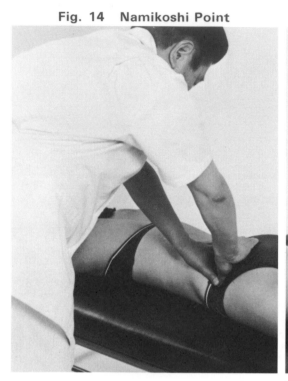

Fig. 15　Posterior Femoral Region

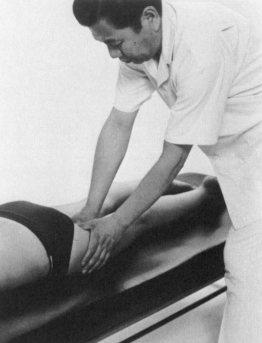

Fig. 16　Posterior Crural Region

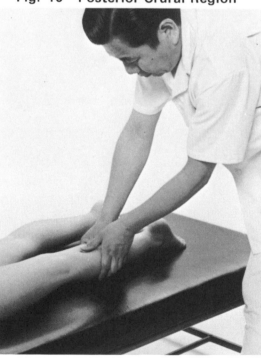

Fig. 17　Both Sides of Posterior Crural Region

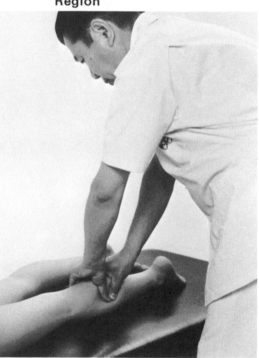

Fig. 18   Calcaneal Tubercle

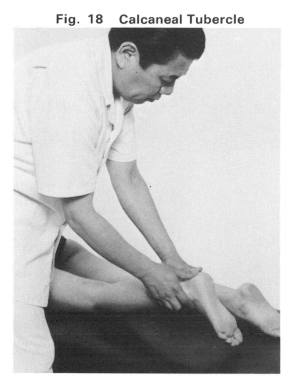

Fig. 19   Lateral and Medial Calcaneus Region

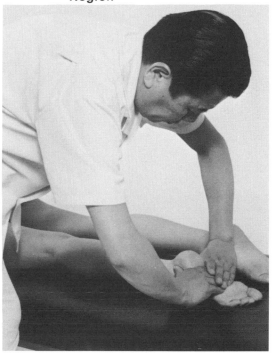
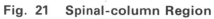

Fig. 20   Plantar Region

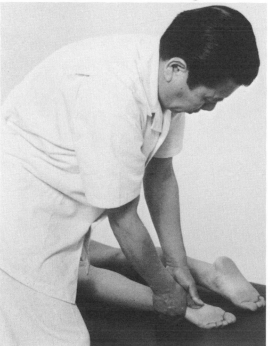

Fig. 21   Spinal-column Region

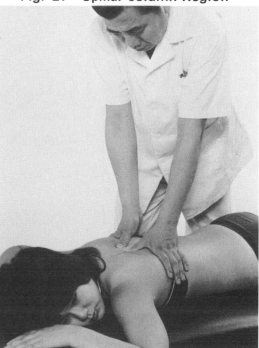

134

Fig. 22   Circular Rotational Pressure on the Scapulae

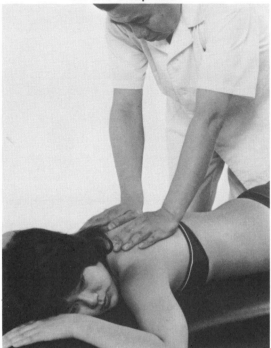

Fig. 23   Adjusting the Transverse Processes

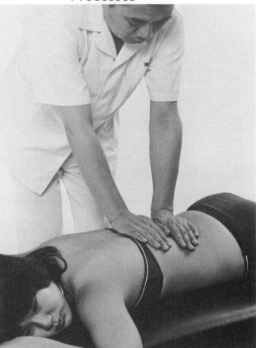

Fig. 24   Adjusting the Spinous Processes

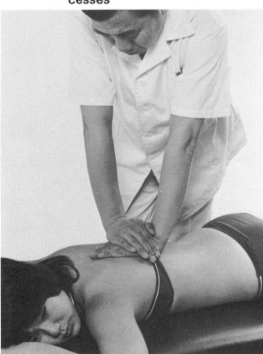

Fig. 25   Downward Stroking with Palm-on-palm Pressure

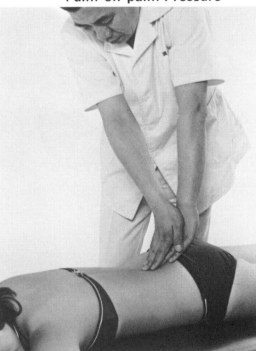

Shiatsu for a Patient Lying in the Supine Position

Fig. 26 Inguinal Region

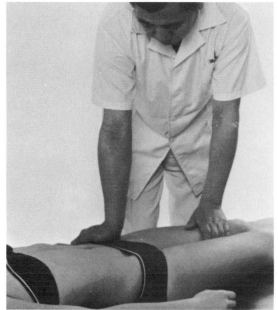

Fig. 27 Anterior Femoral Region

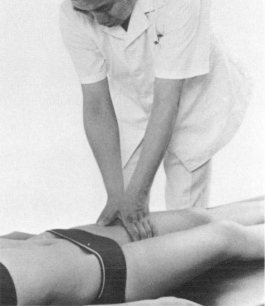

Fig. 28 Medial Femoral Region

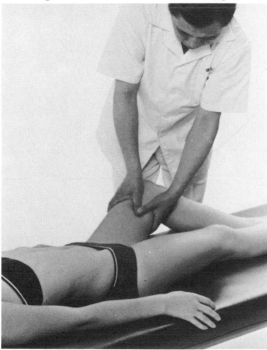

Fig. 29 Lateral Femoral Region

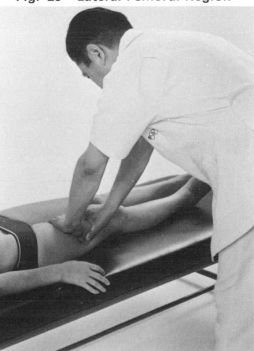

Fig. 30 Patellar Region

Fig. 31 Lateral Crural Region

Fig. 32 Tarsal Region

Fig. 33 Dorsal Region

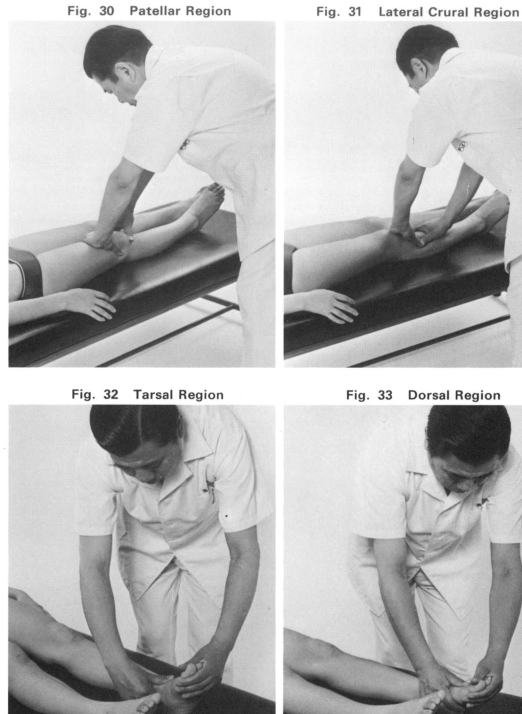

Fig. 34 Digital Region

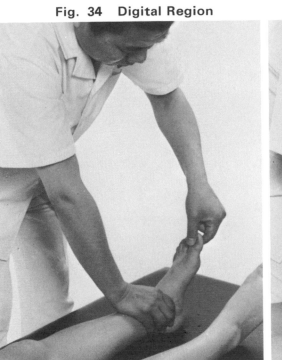

Fig. 35 Plantar Dorsiflexion

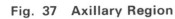

Fig. 36 Extension of the Leg

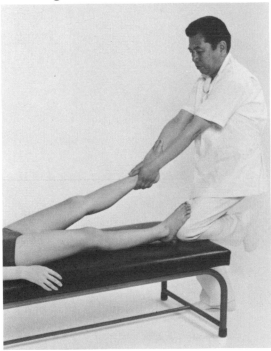

Fig. 37 Axillary Region

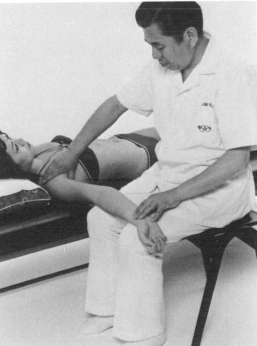

138

Fig. 38   Medial Brachial Region

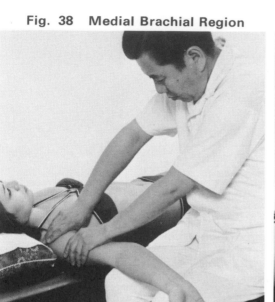

Fig. 39   Cubital Fossa

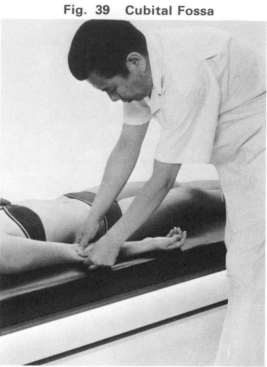

Fig. 40   Medial Antebrachial Region

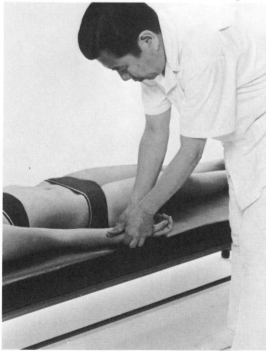

Fig. 41   Extension of the Arm (1)

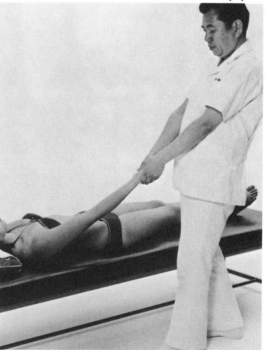

Fig. 42 Extension of the Arm (2)

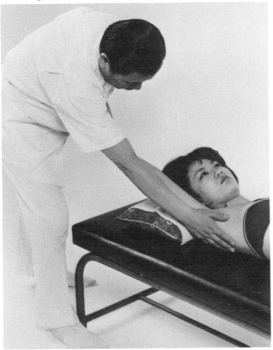

Fig. 43 Extension of the Arm (3)

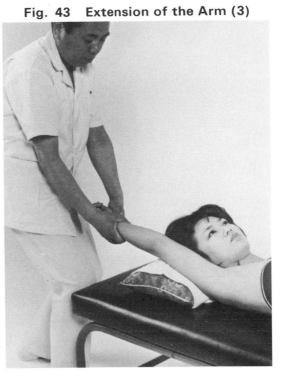

Fig. 44 Extension of the Arm (4)

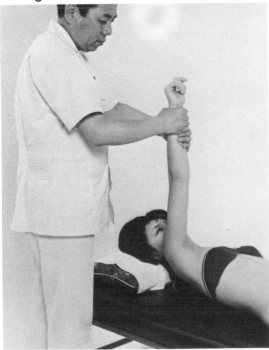

Fig. 45 Extension of the Arm (5)

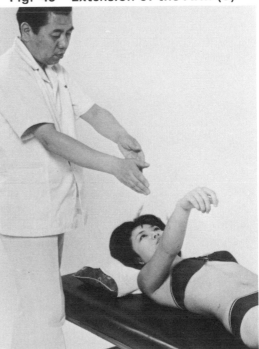

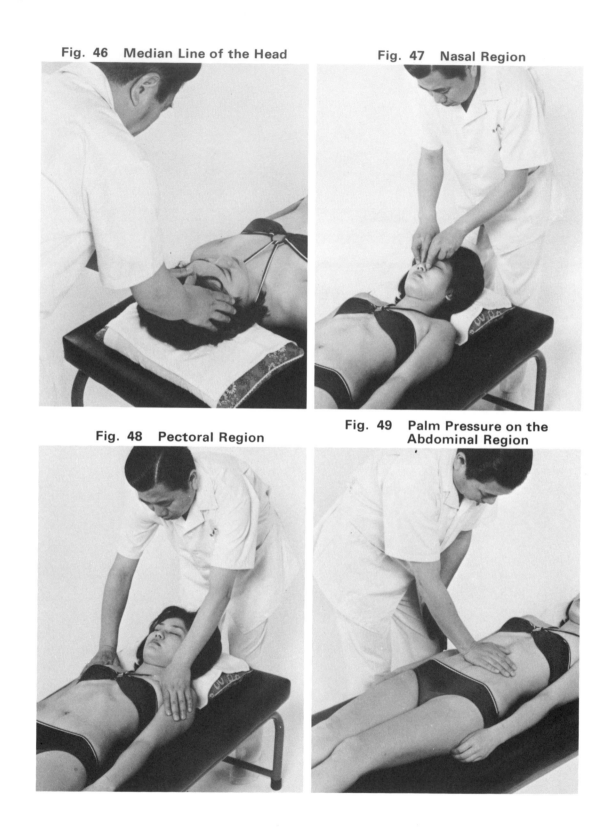

Fig. 46   Median Line of the Head

Fig. 47   Nasal Region

Fig. 48   Pectoral Region

Fig. 49   Palm Pressure on the Abdominal Region

Fig. 50 Two-thumbs Pressure on the Abdominal Region

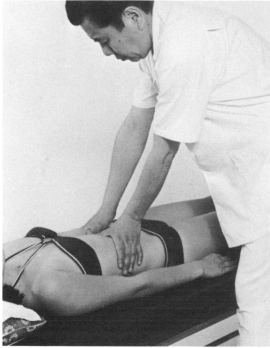

Fig. 51 Rippling Palm Pressure

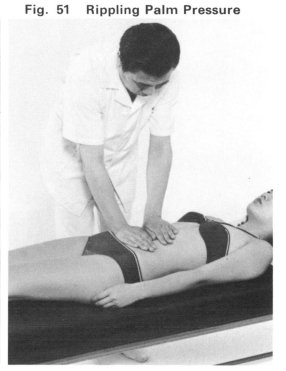

Fig. 52 Circular Palm Pressure

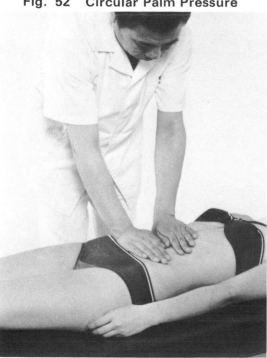

Fig. 53 Upward Kneading of the Spinal-column Region

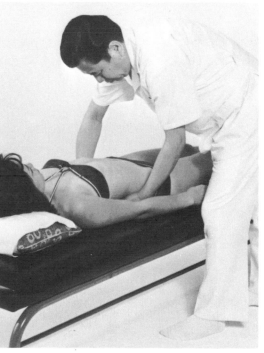

**Fig. 54   Upward Pulling Pressure on the Lateral Abdom-
 inal Region**

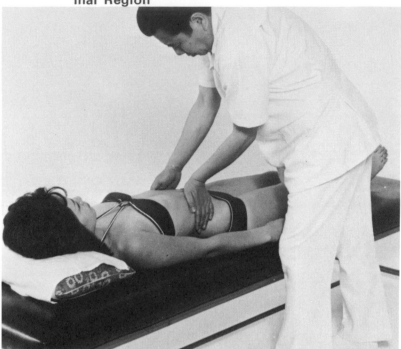

**Fig. 55   Crossed Hand-on-hand Pressure on the Abdom-
inal Region**

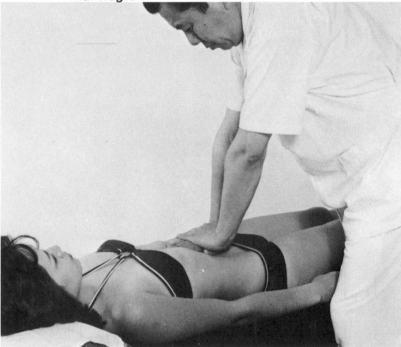

Chapter 4

Therapy for a Kneeling Patient

Shiatsu for a Patient Kneeling on Both Knees (*Seiza* position)

Operation 1: Anterior Cervical Region

The patient kneels on both knees, holding the trunk straight and relaxing neck and suprascapular region. (This is the formal Japanese kneeling position known as *seiza*.) Kneeling on both knees to the left and slightly in front of the patient, the therapist presses his right thumb against point 1 on the left of the patient's anterior cervical region (see p. 63), where the carotid sinus is and where he can feel the pulse of the common carotid artery. He then presses with his right thumb three seconds each on the four points leading downward along this artery to a position beside the thyroid gland and in front of the clavicle. Pressure is applied gently, and the treatment is repeated three times. When treatment on the left side is finished, the therapist moves to a similar position at the patient's right front and repeats the same treatment with the left thumb on the four points on the right anterior cervical region.

Fig. 1

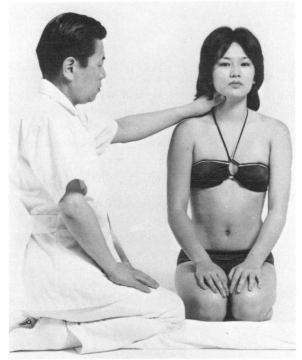

Fig. 2

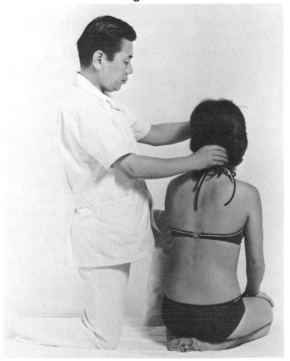

Operation 2: Lateral Cervical Region

The therapist returns to the patient's left side and kneels on his right knee with his left knee raised. Lightly supporting the patient's forehead with his left palm, he treats the left and right sides of the left lateral cervical region with widespread thumb (on the left side) and four fingers (on the right side) of his right hand. Beginning with point 1 (see p. 64) and ending with point 3 at the neck juncture, he presses the points, gradually increasing pressure, for three seconds each and repeats the therapy three times (Fig. 2). Care must be taken that the pressure exerted by the thumb and that exerted by the four fingers are equal.

Operation 3: Medulla Oblongata

With his left palm still supporting the patient's forehead, remaining in the posture employed in operation 2, the therapist presses his right thumb against the region of the medulla oblongata (see p. 65), in the center of the nuchal fossa. He wraps the four fingers of his right hand around the patient's right lateral cervical region for support. The right thumb is pointed upward and through the head toward the patient's glabella, and pressure is applied gradually (Fig. 3). Pressure lasts for five seconds per point, and the therapy is repeated three times. To ensure the pressure's reaching the medulla oblongata, at the first application, the therapist has the patient lean her head forward to an angle of about thirty degrees. Then gradually through the second, third, fourth, and fifth applications, he has her lean her head backward until, at the conclusion of the fifth application, it is tilted in that direction to an angle of about thirty degrees.

Operation 4: Posterior Cervical Region

Employing a method like the one used in operation 3, pressing both the right and left sides of the lateral cervical region, the therapist treats the right and left sides of the posterior cervical region simultaneously with the thumb and four fingers of his right hand (Fig. 4). The three points

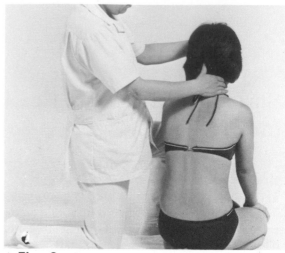

▲ Fig. 3

Fig. 4 ▼

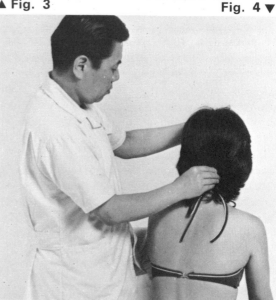

are located on the right and left sides of the rear of the neck (see p. 65). Pressure is a thrust directed to pass through the head and to the face. It lasts for three seconds per point, and therapy is repeated three times.

Operation 5: Temporal Region

Rising, the therapist moves behind the patient and, crouching slightly, stands with feet slightly apart and firm on the floor. Fingers forward and held together, he places the palms of his hands on the right and left sides of the patient's temporal region. He spreads his elbows directly to the side so that his wrists bend at right angles and exerts pressure straight from the sides. When the pressure reaches a suitable intensity, he holds it for a short time (Fig. 5) then quietly relaxes. This is done once for ten seconds.

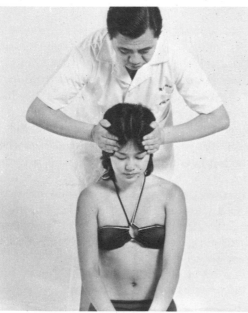

Fig. 5

Operation 6: Suprascapular Region

The therapist stands straight and, with feet still slightly apart, leans his trunk slightly forward and puts his thumbs on the right and left suprascapular points (see p. 66). The four fingers of each hand are pointed forward and opened to form right angles with the thumbs. They are placed lightly for support on the patient's pectoral region. He then applies pressure simultaneously with both thumbs. It is directed toward the center of the trunk at the height of the diaphragm (Fig. 6). Pressure with right and left thumbs must be equal and must result from a natural application of force from the fully outstretched arms. It is applied for five seconds per point, and therapy is repeated three times.

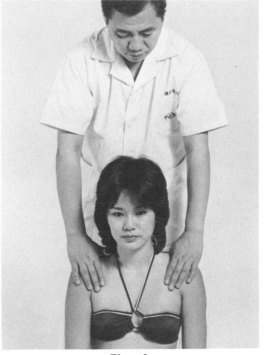

Fig. 6

Operation 7: Interscapular Region

The therapist remains in the same position, but shiatsu shifts from the suprascapular to the interscapular region. The thumbs and four aligned fingers of each hand are spread as far apart as possible. The fingers are placed on the suprascapular region; and the thumbs, pointed downward, are placed on the first right and left interscapular points (see p. 67). Beginning with the left thumb, the therapist applies pressure for three seconds each, alternately with right and left thumbs on the two rows of five interscapular points (Figs. 7 through 9). The therapy is repeated three times. The four fingers of each hand are used to provide firm support so that the thumbs can exert full pressure. Using the principle of the lever, he presses with full arms and body, not with thumbs alone. It is important that right and left pressure exertions be balanced.

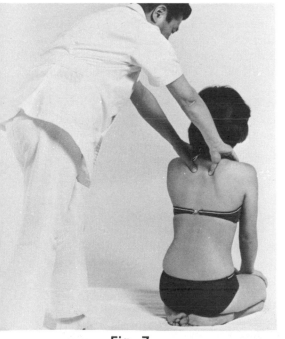

Fig. 7

► **Fig. 8**

Fig. 9

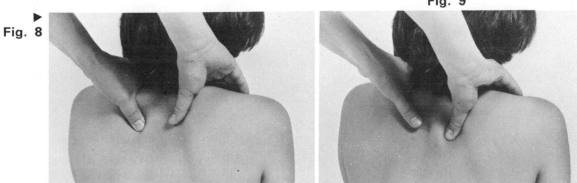

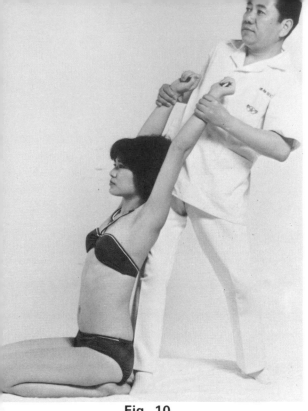

Fig. 10

Operation 8: Extending the Trunk

The therapist takes both of the patient's wrists in his hands and, raising her arms above her head, presses the outer side of the lower part of his right leg against her spinal column as a support. He must turn the toes of his right foot to the side to prevent his knee from coming into contact with her spine. As he pulls her arms upward, he causes her to lean her trunk backward (Fig. 10). The first time, he executes the therapy lightly as a warm-up. The second time, he causes her to lean as far backward as she can—until her face is turned upward—as he pulls her arms. When she has bent fully, he allows her to return to her original position as he pushes both of her arms free and forward (Fig. 11).

Operation 9: Upward and Downward Flexion of the Shoulder Joints

Next, the patient relaxes her shoulders and trunk. The therapist grips her shoulders at the deltoid muscles; his hands should enfold the rounded contour of the shoulders. He raises the shoulders (Fig. 12) as far as possible then suddenly releases them. The shoulders return naturally to their normal position (Fig. 13). This therapy is repeated three times.

Fig. 12   **Fig. 13**

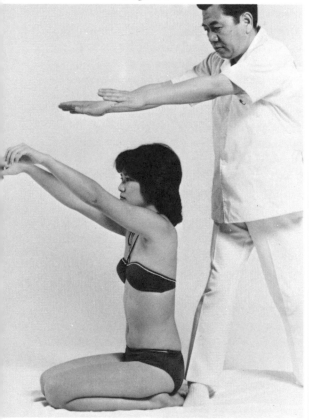

Fig. 11

Fig. 14

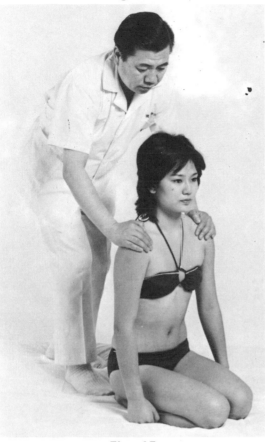

Fig. 15

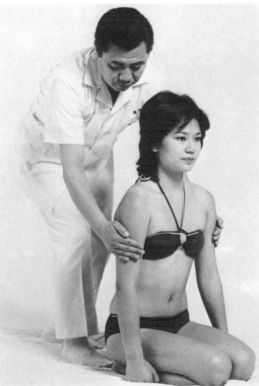

Operation 10: Downward Stroking of the Shoulders and Spinal Column

In the same position, the therapist presses his palms—fingers pointed forward—on the patient's shoulders at the deltoid muscles and quickly strokes both lateral brachial regions downward (Figs. 14 and 15). This therapy is repeated twice.

Then, moving to her left side and facing right, he places his left palm lightly on the patient's left shoulder for support. He puts his right palm—fingers pointed downward—immediately below the vertebral prominence—spinous process of the seventh cervical vertebra—and quickly strokes the spinal column downward to the sacrum twice (Figs 16 and 17).

This concludes the course of therapy for a patient in the *seiza*, or formal kneeling position.

Fig. 16

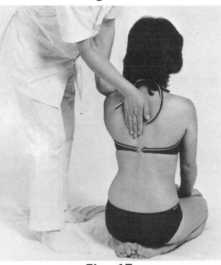

Fig. 17

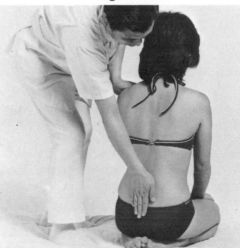

Shiatsu for a Patient Seated Upright in a Chair

Operation 1: Anterior Cervical Region

The patient sits relaxed, trunk straight, in a chair and places both palms lightly on her knees. Standing at the patient's left side and facing sideward, without bending his body, the therapist presses each of the four left anterior cervical points (see p. 63) for three seconds and repeats the therapy three times. The four fingers of the right hand are placed against the patient's posterior cervical region as a support. When treatment of the left side has ended, the therapist moves to the patient's right side and carries out the same treatment on her right anterior cervical region with his left thumb (Fig. 18).

Operation 2: Lateral Cervical Region

Returning to the patient's left side, the therapist assumes the posture he was in at the opening of operation 1. Placing his left palm lightly on the patient's forehead as support, he carries out therapy with his right hand on her lateral cervical region. He spreads the aligned four fingers wide from the thumb of his right hand and puts his hand—thumb on the left side and fingers on the right side—immediately below the mastoid process (Fig. 19). This is the first of the three lateral cervical points. Beginning with it and moving downward to the others, he presses the right and left lateral cervical points simultaneously (Fig. 64) for three seconds each and repeats the therapy three times. Pressure exerted on the right and the left points must be equal.

Operation 3: Medulla Oblongata

Remaining in the position he was in for operation 2, the therapist treats the medulla-oblongata region (see p. 65). His left palm remains on the patient's forehead. With the tip turned upward, he presses the digital ball of his right thumb against the patient's medulla-oblongata region. The other four fingers of the right hand wrap

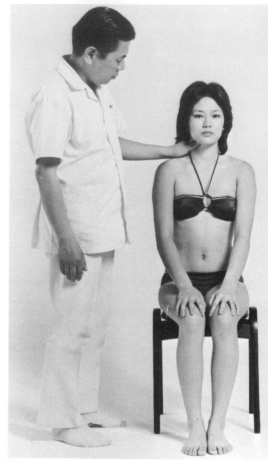

Fig. 18

lightly around the right lateral cervical region as support. While applying pressure, first he has the patient lean her head slightly forward. Gradually he has her raise it and lean it rearward. This slow movement of the head enables the pressure to penetrate easily. Pressure should be directed to the glabella and should be increased gradually. It is applied for five seconds to the point and is repeated three times.

Operation 4: Posterior Cervical Region

Remaining in the same posture, taking the points to the right and left of the medulla oblongata as points 1, the therapist, presses the posterior cervical points (see p. 65) simultaneously: thumb on the left line of points and four fingers on the right line. The pressure is a thrust directed toward the center of the patient's face. Pressure is applied for three seconds per point. The therapy always starts with the uppermost point and moves downward. It is repeated three times.

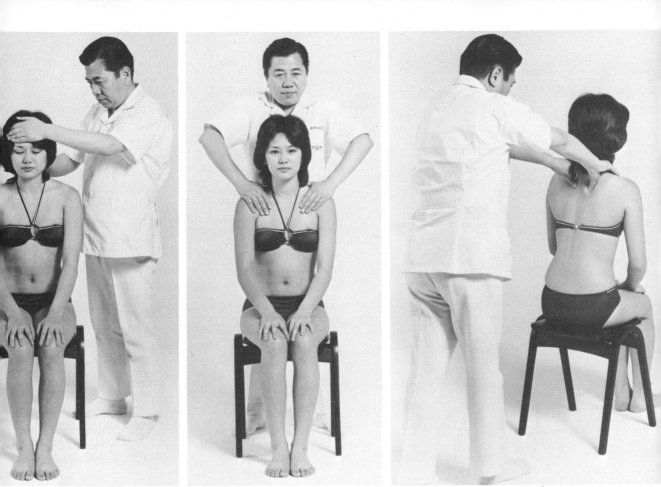

Fig. 19   Fig. 20   Fig. 21

Operation 5: Suprascapular Region

Moving behind the patient, the therapist stands close enough to touch her body with his own body. Extending his elbows to the sides, he places his thumbs on the patient's suprascapular points (see p. 66). The four fingers of each hand—directed forward—are placed for support on the patient's chest. Putting the full weight of his body on them. The therapist directs the pressure toward the center of the trunk at the height of the spinous process of the seventh thoracic vertebra and on a line with the inferior angles of the scapulae. It lasts for five seconds and is repeated three times (Fig. 20).

Operation 6: Interscapular Region

Standing in the position assumed in operation 5, but with one leg pulled to the rear, the therapist puts his thumbs on the first right and left interscapular points (see p. 67) and places the four fingers of his hands on the patient's suprascapular regions for support (Fig. 21). Without break-

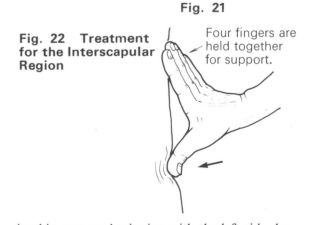

Fig. 22   Treatment for the Interscapular Region

Four fingers are held together for support.

ing his posture, beginning with the left side, he presses first right then left on the two rows of five interscapular points for three seconds per point. The therapy is repeated three times. As the pressure applications move downward, the fingers of both hands, held together and pointed in the direction of the suprascapular regions, move down the patient's back (Fig. 22). These fingers serve to make possible pressure applications based on the principle of the lever.

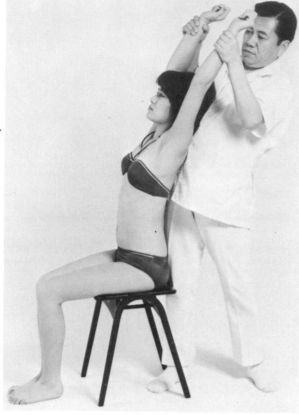

Fig. 23

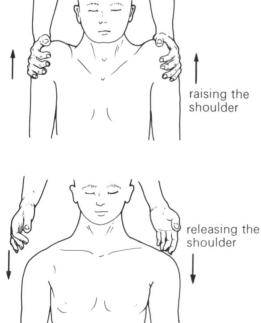

Fig. 24 Upward and Downward Flexion of the Shoulder Joints

raising the
shoulder

releasing the
shoulder

Operation 7: Extending the Trunk

Remaining in the same posture as for operation 6 and pressing the right side of his trunk against the patient's back, the therapist grips both of the patient's wrists and raises her arms above her head. Leaning his own trunk rearward, the therapist pulls the patient's arms and causes her to extend her trunk and stretch her spinal column (Fig. 23). The first time the exercise is performed, it should be only a light warm-up for the second time, which involves a full extension of the patient's trunk. When the patient's body is fully extended, the therapist releases the hands with a forward push.

Operation 8: Upward and Downward Flexion of the Shoulder Joints

The patient thoroughly relaxes her shoulders. Bringing his feet together again, the therapist wraps his hands around the patient's shoulders at the position of the deltoid muscles. After raising both shoulders simultaneously, he releases his hands (Fig. 24). The patient must not tense her shoulders at this time but must allow them to fall naturally into their normal positions. This therapy is repeated three times.

To conclude the treatment for a patient in the seated position, the therapist places his hands on the shoulders. His fingers and thumbs are held together on the outsides of the shoulders at the location of the deltoid muscles. Simultaneously and quickly with both palms, he strokes the patient's shoulders downward.

Fig. 25 Stroking the Shoulders

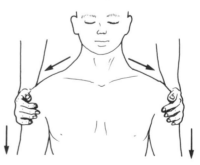

Chapter 5

Self-administered Shiatsu

This chapter shows how self-administered shiatsu serves two highly important functions. First, since use of the hands and fingers, correct selection of pressure application methods, and all basic pressure points must be learned with the whole body and not with the mind alone, using one's own body as practice material makes it easier and faster to master the basics needed to enable a person to perform shiatsu on others. Second, it helps the individual know from daily treatment what parts of his own body are in good condition and what parts require attention, lets him know how to treat the ailing parts, prevents development of illness, and thus sets up a health-conditioning program that is in the fullest sense for and by one's self.

It is especially important to encourage children, even those as young as lower-grade primary-school pupils, to develop the habit of carrying out a self-administered shiatsu program daily, because it can help stimulate physical improvement and greater strength at this time of rapid growth. Perhaps the most important aspect of this program for children is the fourth operation for the face. Shiatsu on the supraorbital and infraorbital regions and the temples and palm pressure on the eyes relieve eye fatigue, promote general eye health, and prevent pseudomyopia. The fifth operation for the face strengthens the gums and thus helps prevent caries and alveolar blennorrhea. Children should be encouraged to spend at least five minutes a day on these two operations.

All of the shiatsu operations discussed in the preceding chapters can be self-administered except those on the right and left interscapular regions.

Cervical Region

Operation 1: Anterior Cervical Region

The anterior cervical region is not only the part of the body where most shiatsu therapy begins, but also the place where some of the most important shiatsu pressure points are located. Obviously, it deserves the most careful therapy. Always begin on the left side and move to the right side when therapy on the left is finished. Kneeling on both knees in the formal *seiza* position, apply pressure with the thumb of one hand. The first point is located at the place where the common carotid artery branches to form the internal and external carotid arteries. On the side of the internal carotid artery is the carotid sinus (see p. 63), where pulse can be felt. Pressing the left thumb—tip pointed upward—on this point, extend your left elbow straight to the side and place the remaining four fingers of your left hand lightly on the front of your neck (Fig. 2). The points for pressure follow the inner edge of the sternocleidomastoid muscle past the thyroid gland and almost to the clavicle. Press each point gently for three seconds and repeat the treatment three times. Pressure must be directed

Fig. 1 Shiatsu Points in the Anterior Cervical Region

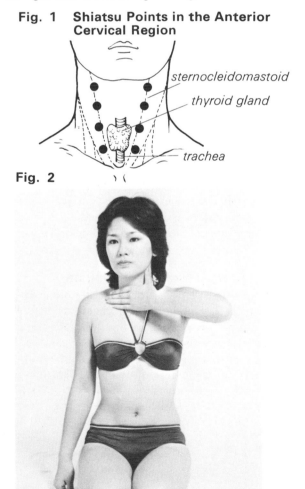

sternocleidomastoid

thyroid gland

trachea

Fig. 2

Fig. 3 Pressure Direction for the Cervical Region

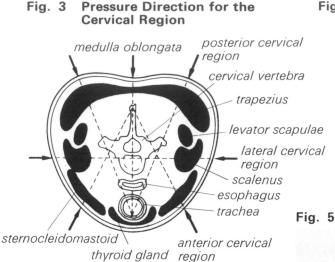

medulla oblongata
posterior cervical region
cervical vertebra
trapezius
levator scapulae
lateral cervical region
scalenus
esophagus
trachea
sternocleidomastoid
thyroid gland
anterior cervical region

Fig. 4 Shiatsu Points in the Lateral Cervical Region

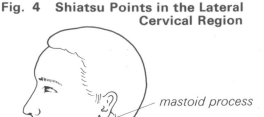

mastoid process
sternocleidomastoid
scalenus
levator scapulae

Fig. 5

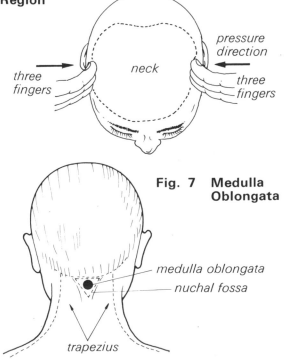

through the neck toward the spinous processes of the cervical vertebrae (Fig. 3). Directing pressure toward the center of the neck constricts the bronchial passage and causes coughing.

Operation 2: Lateral Cervical Region

Both lateral cervical regions are treated simultaneously with the joined index, middle, and ring fingers of both hands. The points for pressure are located from immediately below the mastoid process to the shoulder (Fig. 4). With both elbows extended straight to the sides, with the three fingers mentioned above, press the points on both sides of the neck three seconds each and repeat the treatment three times (Fig. 5). Pressure applied on one side of the cervical region must be directed to the corresponding point on the opposite side of the cervical region (Figs. 3 and 6).

Operation 3: Medulla Oblongata

The pressure point for the medulla oblongata is located in the middle of the nuchal fossa between the occipital bone and the first cervical vertebra (Fig. 7). Place the digital ball of the right middle finger on that point; then put the digital ball of the left middle finger on top of the right middle finger. Extend both elbows straight to the sides (Fig. 8). Incline your head thirty degrees to the front and begin applying pressure on the medulla-

Fig. 6 Pressure Direction for the Lateral Cervical Region

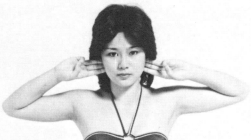

three fingers
neck
pressure direction
three fingers

Fig. 7 Medulla Oblongata

medulla oblongata
nuchal fossa
trapezius

Fig. 8

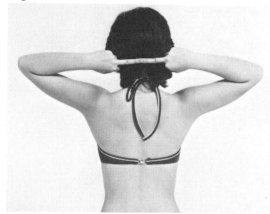

Fig. 10   Shiatsu points in the Posterior Cervical Region

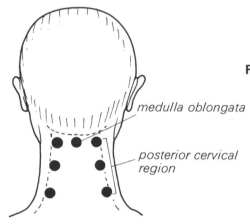

oblongata point. Gradually increase pressure as you bring your head to a vertical position and then incline it thirty degrees to the rear. Pressure should be directed to the glabella (Fig. 9). One application—from forward inclination of thirty degrees to rearward inclination of thirty degrees—lasts five seconds. Repeat three times.

Fig. 9   Pressure Direction for the Medulla Oblongata

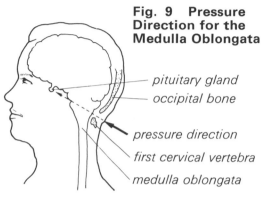

Fig. 11   Pressure Direction for the Posterior Cervical Region

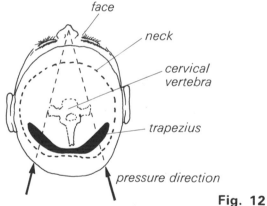

Operation 4: Posterior Cervical Region

The operation by means of which three fingers are used to press the three points (Fig. 10) on either side of the posterior cervical region is like the one used in operation 2. Place the ring fingers on the first points, which are directly beside the point for the medulla oblongata. The index and middle fingers of each hand are aligned naturally with the right fingers. Pressure is directed horizontally toward the median line of the face and is applied first on the uppermost of the three points on each side and then down to the other points. It is applied simultaneously on the right and left sides, three seconds for each point. Therapy is repeated three times (Fig. 12). When you are treating the third point, the index finger should come to the height of the seventh cervical vertebra.

Fig. 12

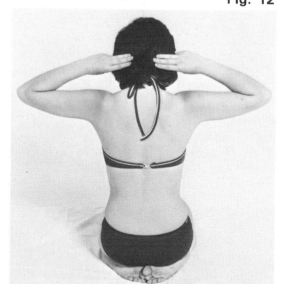

Head

Fig. 13 Median Line on the Head

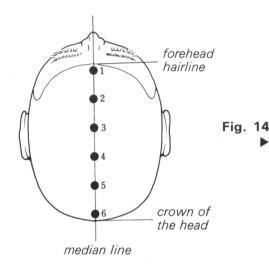

forehead
hairline

crown of
the head

median line

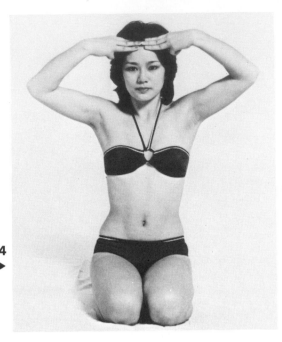

Fig. 14
▶

Operation 1: Median Line

The six points for treatment in this region are located along the median line of the skull from the forehead hairline to the crown of the head. Pressure is applied with the index, middle, and ring fingers of the right hand on top of which are placed the index, middle, and ring fingers of the left hand. It lasts for three seconds for each point, and treatment is repeated three times (Fig. 14). Pressure must be applied at right angles to the surface of the head on all six points (Fig. 15).

Fig. 15 Pressure Direction for the Median Line

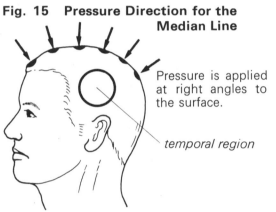

Pressure is applied at right angles to the surface.

temporal region

Fig. 16 Operation for the Median Line

Pressure is directed vertically straight down.

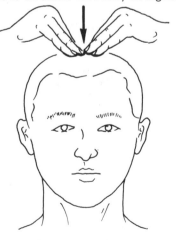

Operation 2: Temporal Region

At the conclusion of the sixth point in operation 1, remove the fingers of the left hand from the fingers of the right hand and place all six—tips touching—on the points for the temporal region, which are arranged three on the left and three on the right of the six points on the median line (eighteen points on each side of the head). Beginning with the index, middle, and ring fingers of each hand, apply pressure simultaneously on the two rows of three points leading from point six on the median line downward toward the temporal hairline (Fig. 17). Pressure must be vertical to the surface of the head all of the time. Repeat with the two rows of three points on each side of the fifth median-line point and so on until you reach the forehead hairline. This treatment is performed once (Fig. 18).

Fig. 17   Shiatsu Points in the Temporal Region

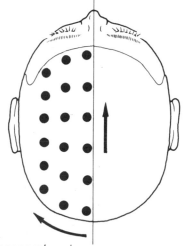

left temporal region

Fig. 18   Treatment for the Temporal Region

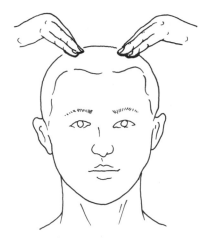

Fig. 19

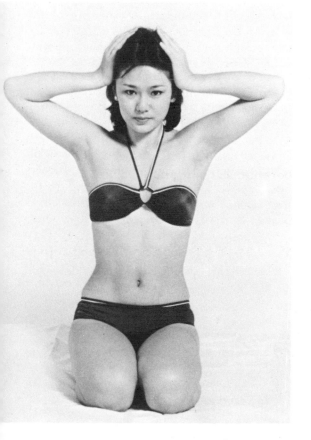

Fig. 20   Palm Pressure on the Temporal Region

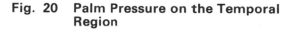

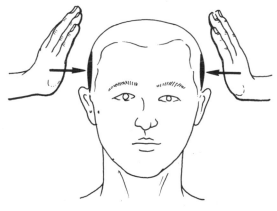

Operation 3: Median Line
Repeat operation 1.

Operation 4: Palm Pressure on the Temporal Region
With the fingers joined and the fingertips pointed upward, press the palms of the hands against the right and left temporal regions (Fig. 15). Extending both elbows straight to the sides, press with balanced, steady force from right and left for ten seconds. The pressure is directed horizontally (Figs. 19 and 20). Vibrational pressure may be used at this time.

Face

Operation 1: Median Line of the Frontal Region

With the index, middle, and ring fingers of the right hand on the bottom and those of the left hand on the top, press the three points on the frontal median line leading upward from just above the glabella (Fig. 21). Pressure is applied for three seconds to a point, and the treatment is repeated three times (Fig. 22).

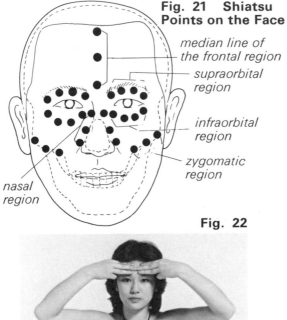

Fig. 21   Shiatsu Points on the Face

median line of the frontal region

supraorbital region

infraorbital region

zygomatic region

nasal region

Fig. 22

Operation 2: Nasal Region

The three points for each side of the nasal region are aligned beside the nose, beginning with the first, located at the inner corner of the eye; moving to the second, beside the nasal bone; and finally reaching the third, immediately adjacent to the wings of the nostrils (Fig. 21). Pressure is applied to the right and left points simultaneously with the digital ball of the index finger of each hand. The digital ball of the middle finger is placed on top of the index finger for stability. Pressure is applied for three seconds to a point, and the treatment is repeated three times (Fig. 23).

Operation 3: Zygomatic Region

The three points for the zygomatic region on each sides of the face lie in an upward line from the sides of the wings of the nostrils to the bases of the ears (Fig. 21). Using the index, middle, and ring fingers of each hand, press in a slightly upward direction simultaneously on each of the points on the right and left sides of the face for three seconds per point. The treatment is repeated three times.

Operation 4: Supra- and Infraorbital Regions and the Temples; Palm-pressure on the Eyeballs

Using the index, middle, and ring fingers of both hands, press each of the four points in the infraorbital region from the inner to the outer corners of both eyes at the same time. Pressure lasts for three seconds on each point, and treatment is repeated three times. Then treat the four points in the supraorbital region in the same way (Figs. 25, and 26). Next, with elbows lowered in front of you, with the digital balls of the index, middle, and ring fingers of each hand—held in a

Fig. 23   **Fig. 24**   **Fig. 25**

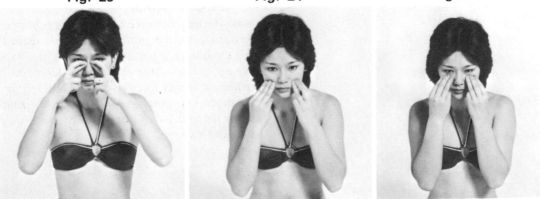

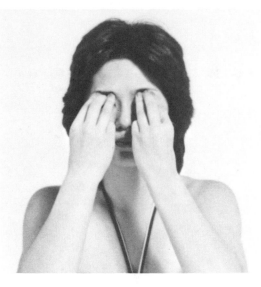

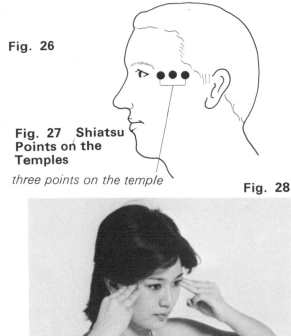

Fig. 26

Fig. 27 Shiatsu Points on the Temples

three points on the temple

Fig. 28

horizontal position—press each of the three temple points leading from the outward corner of the eye to the base of the ear (Fig. 27). Pressure on each point lasts for three seconds, and treatment is repeated three times (Fig. 28). When treatment of the temples is completed, placing the palms of the right and left hands lightly on the eyeballs—fingers pointed upward—press gently on both eyes simultaneously for ten seconds.

Operation 5: Gums
Treatment begins with the mandibular gums and then continues on the maxillary gums (Fig. 29).

Fig. 29 Shiatsu Points on the Gums

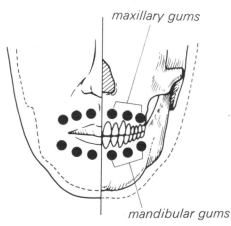

maxillary gums

mandibular gums

The three points for the mandible on each side of the face begin at the median line and follow a line leading to the outer corner of the mouth (Fig. 29). Pressure is applied simultaneously to the points on both sides with the index, middle, and ring fingers of each hand. The ring finger comes into direct contact with each point. Pressure lasts for three seconds per point, and treatment is repeated three times (Fig. 30). At the conclusion of treatment of the mandibular gums, treat the maxillary gums in the same way.

Operation 6: Risorius Muscles at the Corners of the Mouth
Three shiatsu points are located along the risorius muscles on each side of the mouth (Fig. 31). Using the index, middle, and ring fingers of both hands and pulling slightly to the outside as you push, apply pressure simultaneously for three seconds to each of the three points on each side of the face. Treatment is repeated three times (Fig. 32).

Fig. 30 Treatment for the Gums

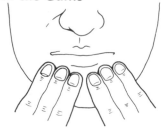

Fig. 31 Shiatsu Points on the Risorius Muscles

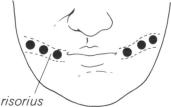

risorius

Fig. 32 Treatment for the Risorius Muscles

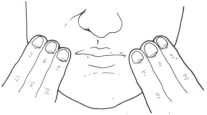

Fig. 33 Suprascapular Region

Fig. 34 Pressure Direction for the Suprascapular Region

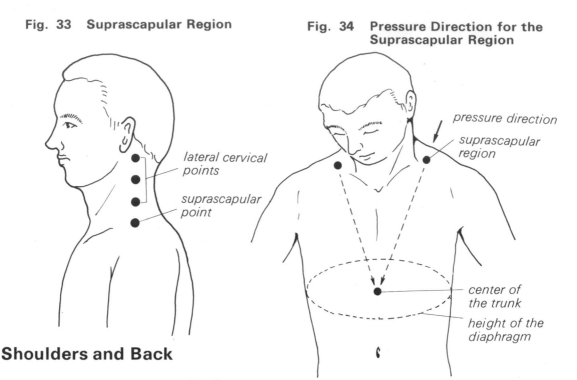

lateral cervical points

suprascapular point

pressure direction

suprascapular region

center of the trunk

height of the diaphragm

Shoulders and Back

Operation 1: Suprascapular Region

Treatment of the suprascapular region must always begin with the left side. With the index, middle, and ring fingers of the right hand, pressure, directed toward the center of the trunk at the height of the epigastric fossa, is applied to the suprascapular point for five seconds (Figs. 33 and 34). Treatment is repeated three times. Then the index, middle, and ring fingers of the left hand are used to perform the same treatment on the right suprascapular point.

Operation 2: Infrascapular and Lumbar Regions

Bringing your arms behind your back and lightly wrapping the four fingers (turned upward) of each hand forward around your side, press the points in the infrascapular region on both sides of the spinal column (Figs. 36 and 37). The first of the ten points on each side of the spine is directly behind the diaphragm. The remainder of the ten extend downward at small intervals to the location of the fifth lumbar vertebra. Pressure is applied to the points on each side of the spine simultaneously with the two thumbs. Leaning the trunk backward enables pressure to penetrate deeply.

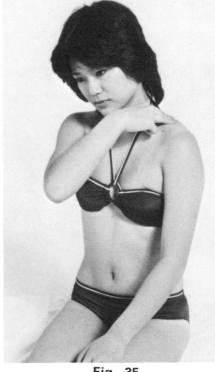

Fig. 35

163

Fig. 36 Infrascapular-lumbar Region

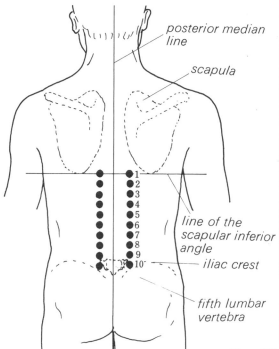

posterior median line

scapula

line of the scapular inferior angle

iliac crest

fifth lumbar vertebra

Fig. 37

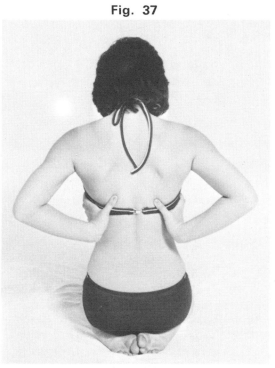

Fig. 38

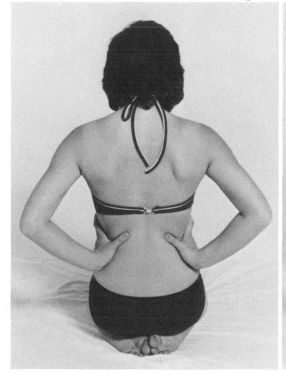

Fig. 39

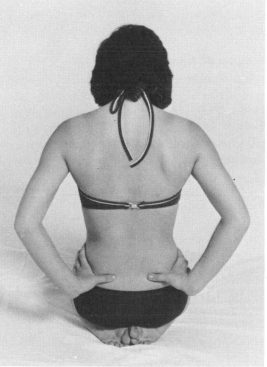

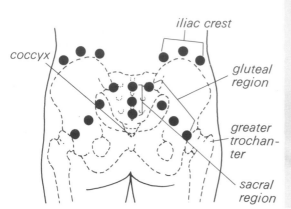

Fig. 40   Shiatsu Points on the Buttocks

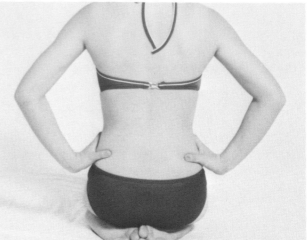

Fig. 41

Operation 3: Iliac Crest

The points for the iliac crest on each side of the hips begin immediately beside the sacroiliac joint and lie along an outward curving line (Fig. 40). There are three to a side. To treat them, the thumbs are oriented in a horizontal line at the same level; and pressure is applied for three seconds to each point. Treatment is repeated three times (Fig. 41). The four fingers of each hand wrap around the lateral abdominal region and move farther as the thumbs move outward to the successive points.

Operation 4: Sacral Region

The three sacral-region points lie along the vertical central line of the sacrum (Fig. 40). With tips brought together, both thumbs are used to press each point for three seconds. Treatment is repeated three times (Fig. 42). Be careful in pressing the last point not to apply pressure to the coccyx.

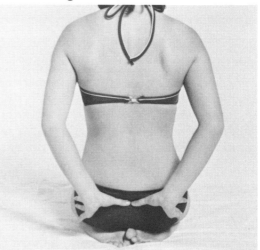

Fig. 42

Legs

This treatment begins with simultaneous shiatsu to the right and left buttocks and then moves first to the left leg and then to the right leg. The explanation is given for the left leg only, since therapy for the right is exactly the same.

Operation 1: Gluteal Region

The two lines of four points for the gluteal region begin on each side of the first of the sacral points and lie along the gluteus maximus muscle, in downward-oriented, outward slanting lines (Fig. 40) and stop immediately short of the greater trochanter. The thumbs are used to press the points on the right and left buttocks simultaneously. Pressure lasts for three seconds per point; the treatment is repeated three times (Fig. 43).

Fig. 43

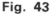

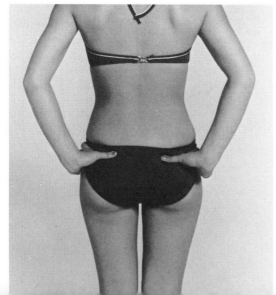

Operation 2: Namikoshi Point

The Namikoshi point is located diagonally below the anterior superior iliac spine and about five centimeters from the spine on a line connecting it with the sacrum (Fig. 44). It is located on the gluteus medius muscle in an area where the superior gluteal nerves are distributed. For this reason, pressure on it passes through the superior gluteal nerves to affect the sciatic nerve. To treat these points, the right and left thumbs are pressed over them—the thumbs are directed toward each other on the same level—and the four fingers of the hands rest on the anterior superior iliac spine for support (Fig. 45). This treatment may be performed in the *seiza* kneeling position; but, if it is more comfortable, you may perform it standing. Pressure should have an upward knead-

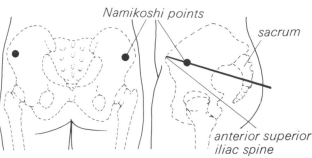

Fig. 44   Namikoshi Point

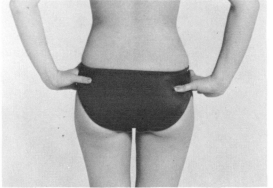

Fig. 45

effect, should be deep and strong, and should be directed toward the greater sciatic notch. It lasts for five seconds and is repeated three times.

Operation 3: Anterior Femoral Region

Sitting with both legs stretched forward and with your left knee slightly raised, press with both thumbs (right thumb on the bottom) on the first anterior femoral point, which is located directly below the anterior superior iliac spine (Fig. 46). The four fingers of both hands wrap around the thigh for support (Fig. 47). Press each of the ten points leading from this position downward to the knee joints three seconds. Repeat the therapy three times (Figs. 48 and 49).

Fig. 46   Ten Points in the Anterior Femoral Region

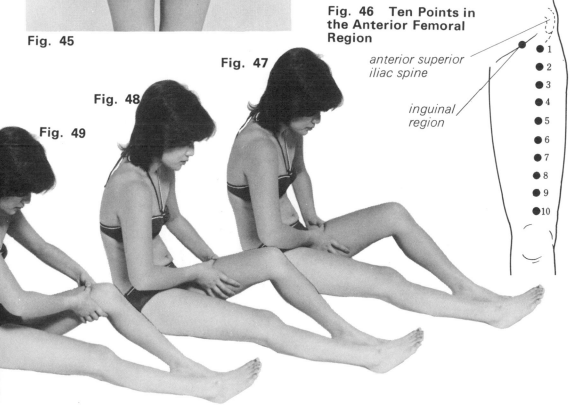

Fig. 47

Fig. 48

Fig. 49

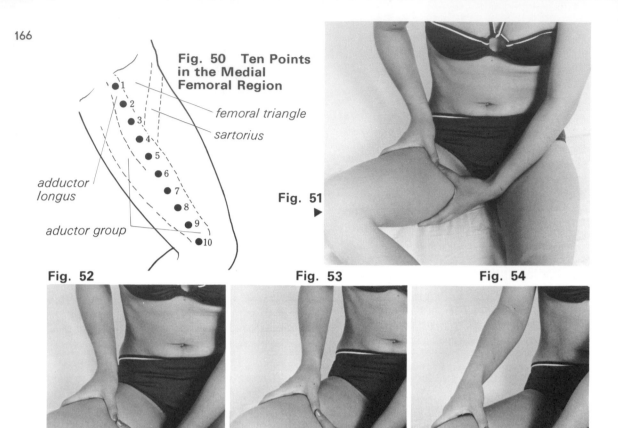

Fig. 50   Ten Points in the Medial Femoral Region

— femoral triangle

— sartorius

adductor longus

aductor group

Fig. 51 ▶

Fig. 52

Fig. 53

Fig. 54

Operation 4: Medial Femoral Region

Bending your left knee outward, bring the sole to a position below the right knee. The ten points for the medial femoral region begin immediately below the pectineus muscle and lie on a line leading to the knee. Pressure is applied in the same manner as in operation 3 to each point for three seconds, and treatment is repeated three times (Figs. 50 through 54).

Operation 5: Lateral Femoral Region

Return your left leg to its original position, then bend it inward so that it lies over your right knee. With both thumbs—outer edges touching— and the four fingers wrapped around the thigh for support, press the ten lateral-femoral points, which begin directly beside the greater trochanter and lie along the femur on a line leading to the knee joint (Fig. 55). Pressure on each point lasts for three seconds, and the treatment is repeated three times (Figs. 56 and 57).

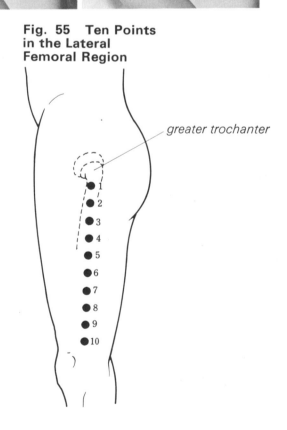

Fig. 55   Ten Points in the Lateral Femoral Region

— greater trochanter

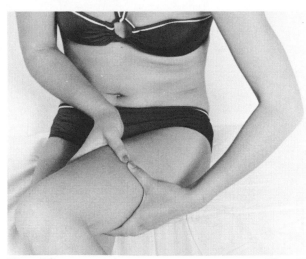

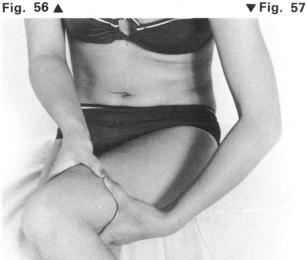

Fig. 56 ▲   ▼ Fig. 57

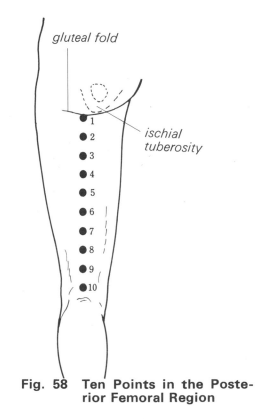

gluteal fold

ischial tuberosity

1
2
3
4
5
6
7
8
9
10

Fig. 58   Ten Points in the Posterior Femoral Region

Fig. 59

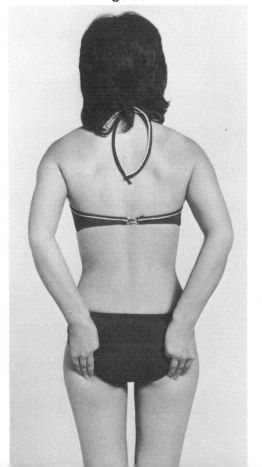

Operation 6: Posterior Femoral Region

The first of the ten points for the posterior femoral region lies in the gluteal fold below the sciatic tuber, and the remaining lie on a line extending downward to the popliteal fossa. It is easier to treat the first points in a standing position. With the index, middle, and ring fingers of each hand, simultaneously press these points for three seconds and repeat the treatment three times. When you have completed this treatment, sit on the floor with your legs outstretched to the front. Raise your left knee high. Put the index, middle, and ring fingers (digital balls) of each hand, fingertips touching, on the second of the ten posterior-femoral points. Wrap your thumbs around the thigh for support. Press on each point from the second to the tenth for three seconds and repeat the therapy three times (Figs. 60 and 61).

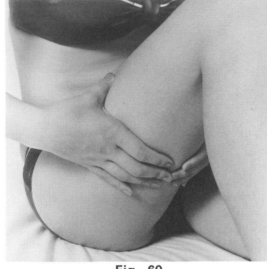

Fig. 60

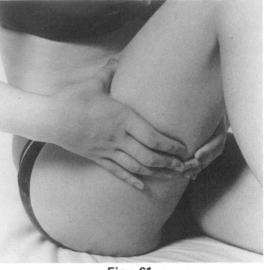

Fig. 61

Operation 7: Patellar Region

Raise your left knee slightly off the floor. With both thumbs—tips touching—press each of the three points below the knee and each of the three points above the knee (Fig. 62) for three seconds. Repeat the treatment three times. In each case, begin with the outer point and move inward and wrap the four fingers of both hands around the knee for support.

Operation 8: Popliteal Fossa

With both thumbs on the side of the knee joint, press the digital balls of the index, middle, and ring fingers of both hands on the first, second, and third of the three points (Fig. 66) across the popliteal fossa, moving from the outside inward. Press each point for three seconds and repeat the treatment three times (Fig. 65).

Fig. 62   Shiatsu Points in the Popliteal Fossa

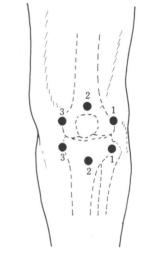

Fig. 63

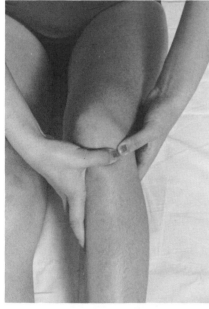

Fig. 64

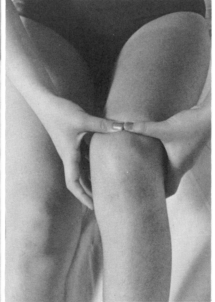

Fig. 65

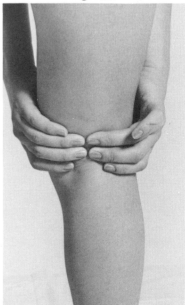

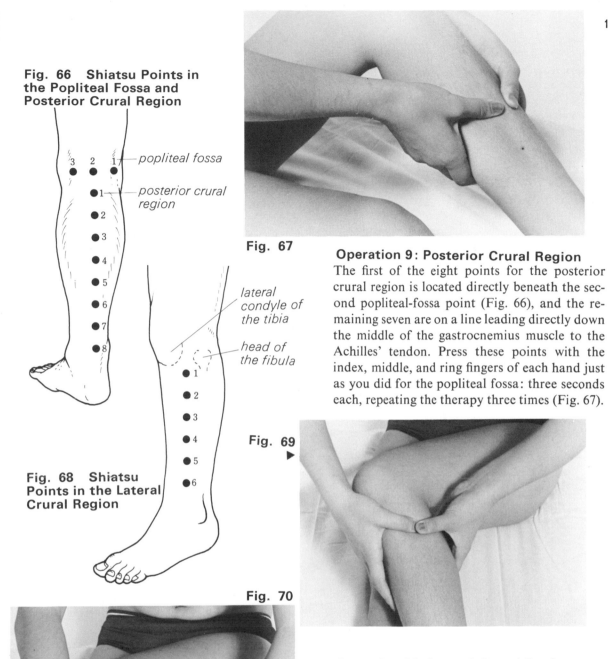

Fig. 66 Shiatsu Points in the Popliteal Fossa and Posterior Crural Region

popliteal fossa

posterior crural region

Fig. 67

lateral condyle of the tibia

head of the fibula

Fig. 69 ▶

Fig. 68 Shiatsu Points in the Lateral Crural Region

Fig. 70

Operation 9: Posterior Crural Region

The first of the eight points for the posterior crural region is located directly beneath the second popliteal-fossa point (Fig. 66), and the remaining seven are on a line leading directly down the middle of the gastrocnemius muscle to the Achilles' tendon. Press these points with the index, middle, and ring fingers of each hand just as you did for the popliteal fossa: three seconds each, repeating the therapy three times (Fig. 67).

Operation 10: Lateral Crural Region

To treat the lateral crural region, bend your left knee inward so that your left leg lies on your right leg. The first of the six points for the lateral crural region is located directly below the lateral condyle of the tibia (Fig. 68). Press it for five seconds firmly with overlapping thumbs; the four fingers of each hand wrap around the leg for support (Fig. 69). Continue to treat the remaining five points which lie between the tibia and the fibula: three seconds for each point, with the treatment repeated three times (Fig. 70).

Operation 11: Tarsal Region

Raising your left knee and pulling your foot toward your trunk, treat the three points of the tarsal region from the lateral to the medial malleolus (Fig. 77). The fingers of the hands are wrapped around the ankle for support, and the thumbs—tips touching—are used to apply pressure for three seconds to each point. The therapy is repeated three times (Figs. 72 through 74).

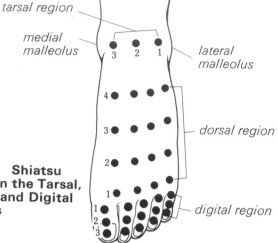

Fig. 71 Shiatsu Points in the Tarsal, Dorsal, and Digital Regions

Fig. 72

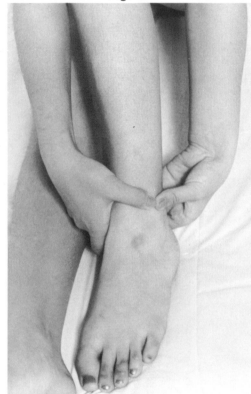

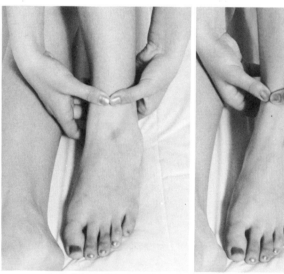

Fig. 73   **Fig. 74**

Fig. 75
▶

Operation 12: Dorsal Region of the Foot (Interosseous Metatarsal Region)

Following operation 11, press with overlapping thumbs on the interosseous metatarsal regions, beginning with the space between the bases of the first and second toes and pressing for three seconds on each of the four points across the dorsal region at the bases of the toes. Then press the remaining three rows of four points. Pressure lasts for three seconds per point; the therapy is performed once (Fig. 75).

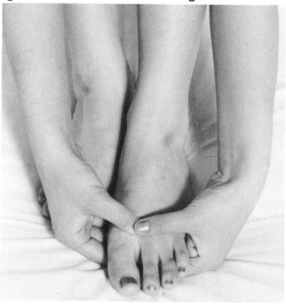

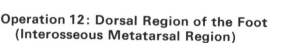

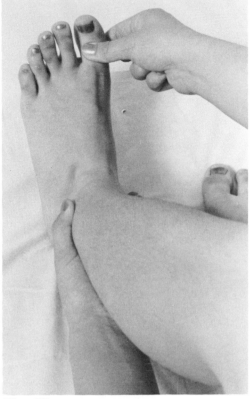

Fig. 76

Operation 13: Digital Region

Bending the ankle upward and holding it in the left hand, with the thumb and index finger of the right hand, from the top, press the dorsal and plantar surfaces of the three points located on the proximal, middle, and distal phalanges of each toe for three seconds each (Figs. 71 and 76). At the distal phalanx of each toe, pull the toe upward as you press. This therapy is performed once.

Operation 14: Plantar Region

Bend the left knee outward and down and turn the sole of the left foot upward. The four plantar-region points are located slightly below the fork of the second and third toes. The second point is directly below that; the third, in the arch; and the fourth, in the middle of the heel (Fig. 77). With both thumbs—either overlapped or with outer edges touching—and with the four fingers wrapped around the dorsal surface of the foot, press each of these points for three seconds and repeat the therapy three times. Complete the treatment by using overlapped thumbs to press the third point strongly three times for five seconds each time (Fig. 81).

Fig. 77 Shiatsu Points in the Plantar Region

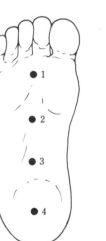

Fig. 78

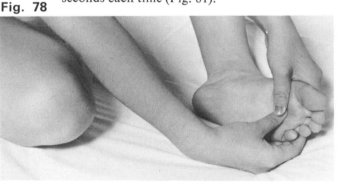

Fig. 79

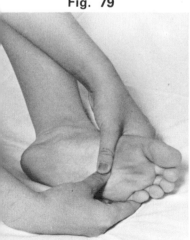

Fig. 80

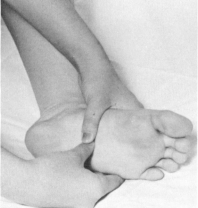

Fig. 81

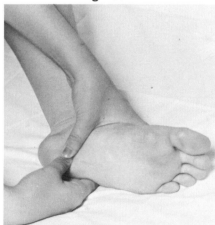

Arms

As was the case in treatment for the legs, explanations are given for the left arm only; the treatment for the right arm is the same.

Operation 1: Axillary Region

Turning the palm of the left hand upward, outstretch the arm to the side. Place the index, middle, and ring fingers of the right hand in the axilla (Fig. 82), with the thumb held against the deltopectoral groove. Press the point with the digital balls of the fingers for five seconds and repeat three times; the pressure is directed toward the suprascapular region (Fig. 83).

Operation 2: Medial Brachial Region

The six points for the medial brachial region are in a straight line from the axilla to the cubital fossa. With the thumb of the right hand—tip turned toward the axilla—and the other four fingers wrapped around the arm, press each of these six points (Fig. 82) for three seconds and repeat the therapy three times (Figs. 84 and 85).

Fig. 82 Shiatsu Points in the Medial Brachial Region

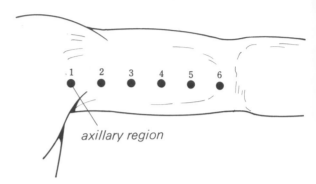

axillary region

Fig. 83

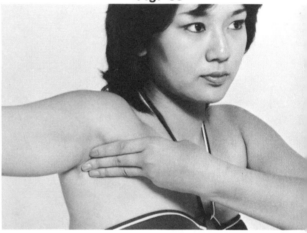

Fig. 84

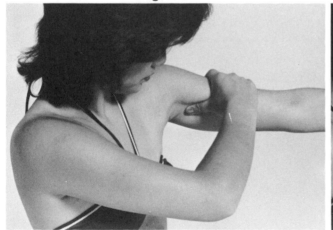

Fig. 85

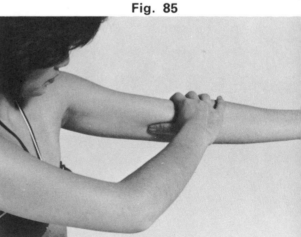

173

Fig. 86 Shiatsu Points in the Cubital Fossa, Medial Antebrachial, Palmar, and Digital Regions

Operation 3: Cubital Fossa

The three cubital-fossa points are located on a line from inner (little-finger) to outer (thumb) side of the fossa (Fig. 86). With the thumb of the right hand—tip pointed upward—and with the other four fingers wrapped around the arm, press each of these points for three seconds and repeat the therapy three times (Figs. 87 through 89).

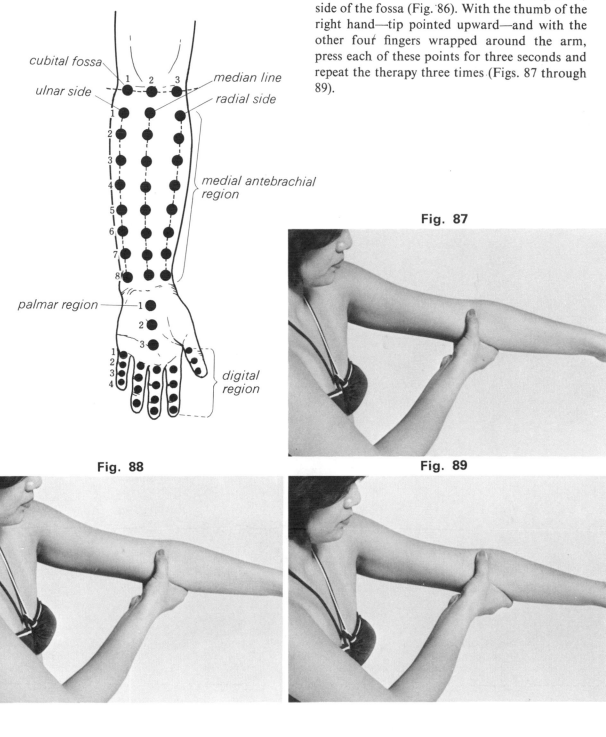

Fig. 87

Fig. 88

Fig. 89

174

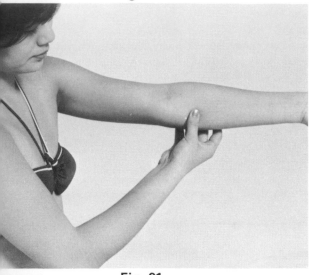

Fig. 90

Operation 4: Medial Antebrachial Region

The twenty-four points for this part of the arm are arranged in eight horizontal rows of three points each moving from the ulnar (little-finger) side to the radial (thumb) side. The vertical rows are directly below the three points in the cubital fossa (Fig. 86). With the right thumb—tip turned upward—press each of these points for three seconds. This therapy is performed once (Figs. 90 through 94).

Operation 5: Deltopectoral Groove

Three points are located along the deltopectoral groove leading downward in a slightly curved

Fig. 91

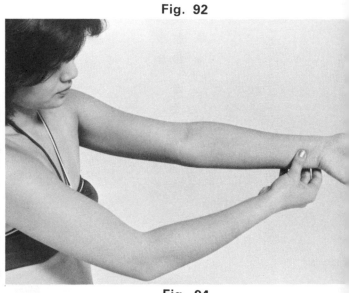

Fig. 92

Fig. 93

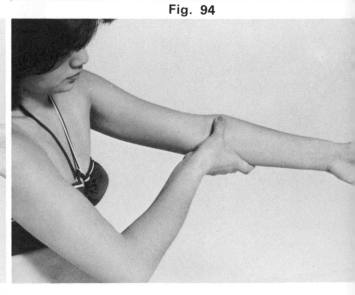

Fig. 94

diagonal line. With the thumb of the right hand —tip pointed diagonally upward—and with the four fingers wrapped around the outer side of the arm, press each point for three seconds. Repeat the therapy three times (Fig. 95).

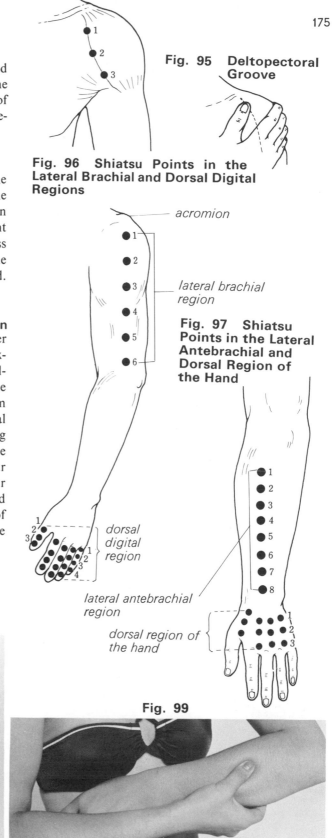

Fig. 95   Deltopectoral Groove

Fig. 96   Shiatsu Points in the Lateral Brachial and Dorsal Digital Regions

acromion

lateral brachial region

Fig. 97   Shiatsu Points in the Lateral Antebrachial and Dorsal Region of the Hand

dorsal digital region

lateral antebrachial region

dorsal region of the hand

Operation 6: Lateral Brachial Region

Turn your arm so that the palm is inward. The six points for this region are located along the center of the deltoid muscle from the acromion to the elbow joint (Fig. 96). With thumb bent around the inside of the arm for support, press each of these points for three seconds with the index, middle, and ring fingers of the right hand. Repeat the therapy three times.

Operation 7: Lateral Antebrachial Region

If you hold all four fingers of your hand together and flex them, you will notice motion of the extensor digitorum communis muscle near the elbow. The place where this motion occurs is the first of the eight points that are on a line from there to the wrist in the lateral antebrachial region. To treat them, bend your elbow to bring your forearm in front of your chest. With the thumb of your right hand—pointed toward your elbow—press the first point. The other four fingers of the right hand are wrapped around the arm for support. Apply pressure to each of the points for three seconds and repeat the therapy three times. (Figs. 98 and 99).

Fig. 98

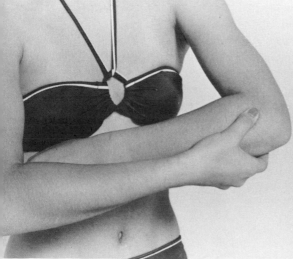

Fig. 99

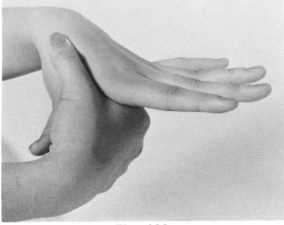

Fig. 100

Fig. 101 Shiatsu Points in the Digital Region

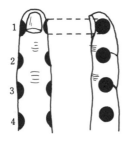

Fig. 102
▶

Fig. 104

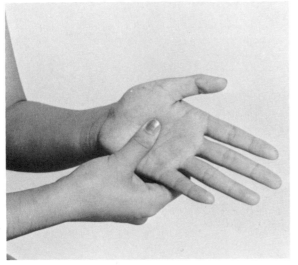

Operation 8: Dorsal Region of the Hand

The interosseous points on the dorsal side of the hand are located between the bones in four lines of three points each moving from the wrist toward the bases of the fingers (Fig. 97). With the right thumb—turned toward the wrist—press each of these points, beginning on the thumb side of the hand, once for three seconds. The four fingers of the right hand wrap around the palm for support (Fig. 100).

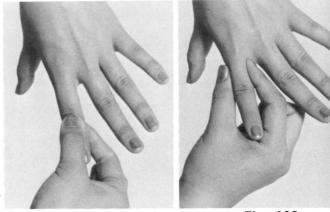

Fig. 103

Operation 9: Digital Region

There are three pressure points on the thumb on a line from the proximal to the distal phalanges. With the thumb and index finger of the right hand, press each point, dorsal and palmar sides, simultaneously, for three seconds. Pull as you apply pressure to the point on the distal phalanx. Next, treat the right and left sides of each point in the same way. At the conclusion of treatment of the thumb, treat the four points on each of the other fingers in the same manner (Figs. 102 and 103).

Operation 10: Palmar Region

There are three pressure points on the median line of the palm: the first is on the heel of the hand, the second in the middle of the palm, and the third at the base of the middle finger (Fig. 86). With the other four fingers wrapped around the dorsal side of the hand for support, press each of these three points with the right thumb for three seconds. Repeat the treatment three times (Fig. 104).

Operation 11: Extension of the Arm

Place the thumb of your right hand in the center of your left palm and wrap the other four fingers around the dorsal side of the left hand. Raise your right hand to shoulder level and pull it forward with your left hand (Fig. 105). This arm extension takes five seconds and is repeated three times.

Chest

Operation 1: Intercostal Region

This treatment is for the pectoralis major muscle and the internal and external intercostal muscles. Press the index, middle, and ring fingers of each hand immediately to the side of the sternal body. Each finger comes between two ribs. Extending your elbows straight to the side, press each of the four intercostal points on the right and left sides of the body simultaneously. There are six horizontal rows of such points on each side. The upper three rows are pressed at one time; then the lower three rows. Pressure lasts for three seconds, and the treatment is performed once. Pressure is applied with a slight outward pull (Figs. 107 and 108).

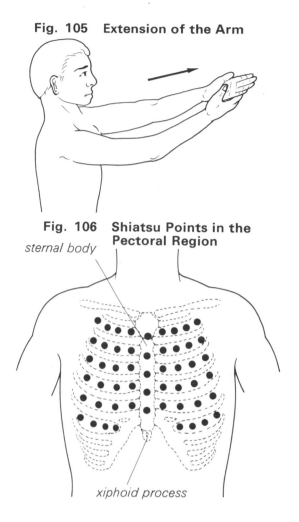

Fig. 105   Extension of the Arm

Fig. 106   Shiatsu Points in the Pectoral Region

sternal body

xiphoid process

Fig. 107

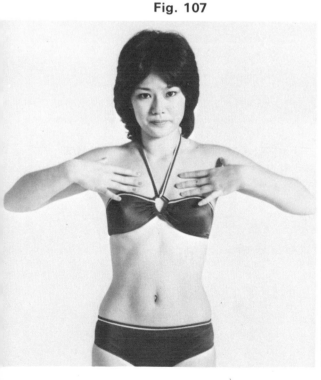

Fig. 108

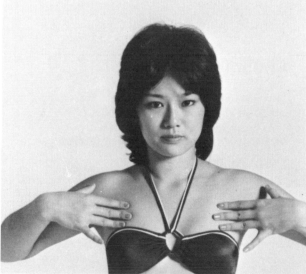

Fig. 109

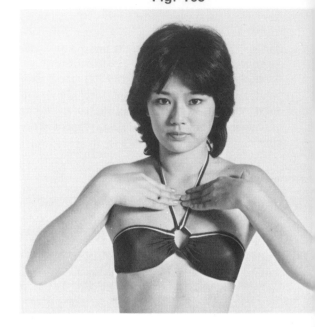

Operation 2: Sternal Region

The five sternal points begin at the top of the sternal body—manubrium—and extend to the xiphoid process (Fig. 106). Using the index, middle, and ring fingers of both hands, tips held together, lightly press each point for three seconds. The therapy is performed once (Fig. 109). Take care to apply no pressure to the xiphoid process.

Operation 3: Circular Rotational Palm Pressure on the Pectoral Region

With fingers directed toward the sternal body, place the palms of your hands on your left and right pectoral regions and extend your elbows straight to the sides. Simultaneously apply outward-rotating palm pressure five times (Fig. 110). When your hands have returned to their original positions at the end of this treatment, turn your fingers toward your diaphragm and slide them rapidly downward across your chest (Fig. 111). Repeat twice. Exhale sharply in synchronization with the rapid downward stroking.

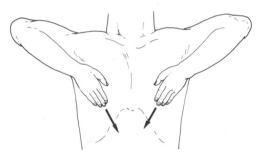

Fig. 111 Downward Stroking Palm Pressure

Fig. 110 Circular Rotational Palm Pressure

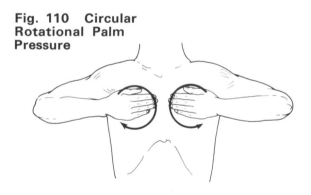

Abdomen

Fig. 112 Nine Points for the Palm-Pressure Series

This therapy may be performed in either the seated or the prone position.

Operation 1: Palm Pressure Series

The first point in this series is located on the diaphragm in the epigastric fossa. The second, third, fourth, fifth, sixth, seventh, eighth, and ninth are arranged on a line that descends toward the pubic region, rises on the right side of the abdomen, and crosses and descends on the left side of the abdomen (Fig. 112). Pressure is applied with both palms, right underneath and left on top, three seconds to a point. The treatment is

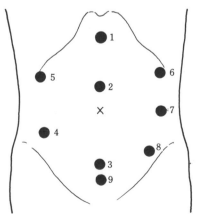

Fig. 113

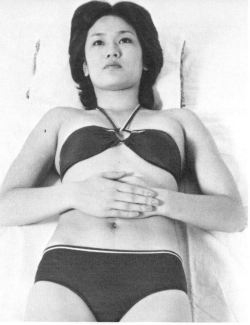

repeated three times. Point 1 is over the stomach, point 2 over the small intestine, point 3 over the bladder, point 4 over the cecum, point 5 over the liver, point 6 over the spleen, point 7 over the descending colon, point 8 over the sigmoid colon, and point 9 over the rectum. Prior to each application of pressure, inhale deeply then gradually increase pressure so that it has a quiet, deeply penetrating effect. Exhale in synchronization with the application (Figs. 113 through 117). When stiffness has been relieved in the abdominal area, these same points may be treated with the index, middle, and ring fingers of both hands—tips touching.

Fig. 114

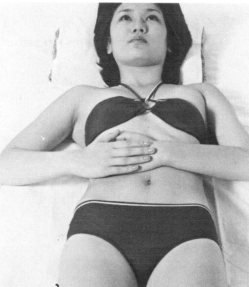

Fig. 115

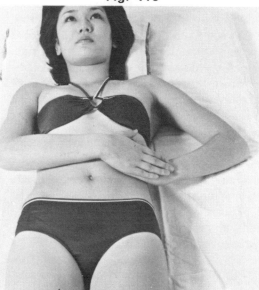

Fig. 116

Fig. 117

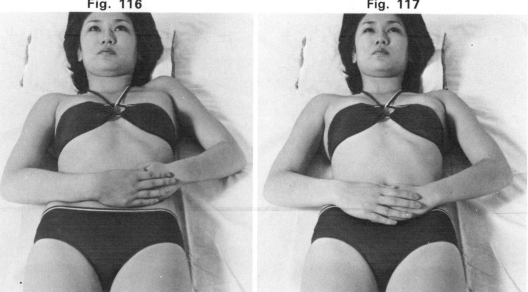

Operation 2: Small-intestine Region

The points for this treatment are located in a circle around the navel. The first is diagonally to the right and above the navel, and the remainder lie on a clockwise circle (Fig. 118). Pressure is applied to each for three seconds with the index, middle, and ring fingers of both hands—tips touching. The treatment is repeated three times.

Operation 3: Region of the Descending and Ascending Colons

Place your right palm over your navel with the fingers of that hand held together and pointed directly to the side in a position over the descending colon. Place the left hand, palm down, over the right hand. It is oriented in the opposite direction. First with the digital balls of the right hand pull the descending colon in the direction of the navel. When you have pulled as far as you can, release and, with the carpus of the hand, push the ascending colon in the direction of the navel (Fig. 119). Repeat this pull and push in a rippling motion ten times. Then, leaving the palms in the same position and pressing with them so that they do not slip, exert circular rotational pressure ten times (Fig. 120). Then exert deep-penetrating vibrational pressure for ten seconds to conclude the self-administered shiatsu treatment (Fig. 121).

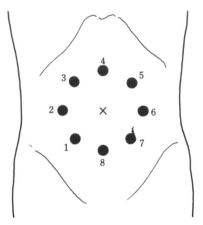

Fig. 118 Shiatsu Points over the Small Intestine

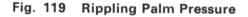

Fig. 119 Rippling Palm Pressure

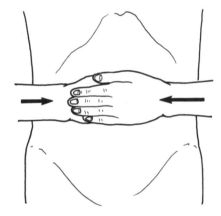

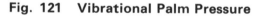

Fig. 120 Circular Rotational Palm Pressure

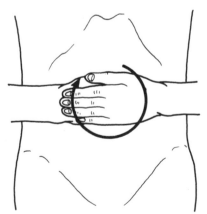

Fig. 121 Vibrational Palm Pressure

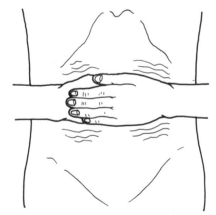

Chapter 6

Treating Specific
Pathological Conditions

The explanations for therapy in cases of specific pathological conditions presume mastery of general techniques. For details, see the preceding chapters.

Circulatory System

1. Cardiac Conditions

Angina pectoris. The condition is caused by coronary arteriosclerosis, bringing about constriction of the coronary artery with obstruction of circulation to the cardiac muscles, which contract spasmodically and inhibit oxygen supply. The agonizing pain in the chest brought on by this condition is called angina pectoris.

Cardiac insufficiency. This may be caused by hypertension, pathological alterations in cardiac muscle accompanying arteriosclerosis, or by excess load on the heart caused by endocarditis or valvular heart disease, which hinder cardiac functioning and make respiration difficult.

Cardiac infarction. A serious angina pectoris paroxysm, this condition causes severe, sudden pain in the area of the sternum, the left pectoral area, and the epigastric fossa. Blood pressure drops, and such shock as cyanosis and respiratory difficulty occur. The condition is dangerous. It is caused by thrombus brought on by severe arteriosclerosis and impediment to blood flow in the coronary artery, with resulting cessation of cardiac function and necrosis.

Shiatsu Therapy

A person who suspects cardiac irregularity should undergo the following shiatsu therapy as an early-phase preventative; should avoid stimulants like coffee, tobacco, and alcohol, should carefully regulate his daily diet, and should try to put his body in good condition.

1. Having the patient lie in the left lateral position, the therapist performs shiatsu treatment on the four points on the anterior cervical region (therapy for rapid action of the heart and pulse), suprascapular region and five points on the left interscapular region (therapy for slow action of the heart and pulse: Figs. 1 and 2). In cardiac patients, stiffness always develops in the profound zones under the area from the second to

Fig. 1

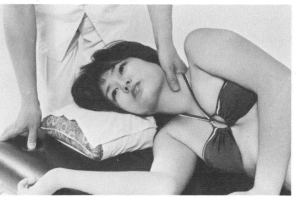

Fig. 2

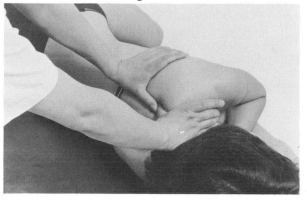
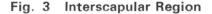

Fig. 3 Interscapular Region

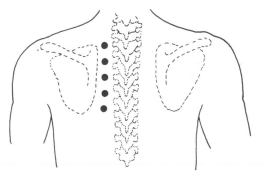

Fig. 4 Medial Surface of the Arm

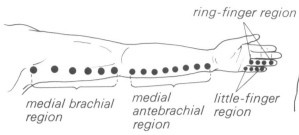

ring-finger region

medial brachial region

medial antebrachial region

little-finger region

Fig. 5 Deltopectoral Groove, Pectoral and Epigastric-fossa Regions

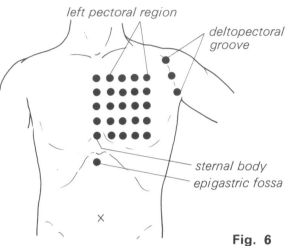

left pectoral region

deltopectoral groove

sternal body

epigastric fossa

the fifth points in the interscapular region (Fig. 3). The therapist must take great care to relieve this tension thoroughly.

2. Having the patient remain in the left lateral position, the therapist raises her left arm directly above her head and carefully treats the three points in the deltopectoral groove, the six points in the medial brachial region from the axilla to the elbow joint, the eight points on the antebrachial ulnar side, and the four points in the dorsal and palmar sides of the little and ring fingers (Fig. 6). Then, with the patient's arm

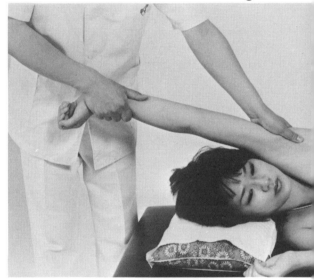

Fig. 6

Fig. 7

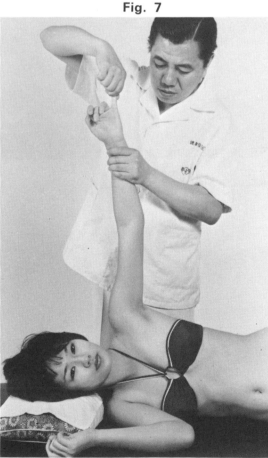

Fig. 8

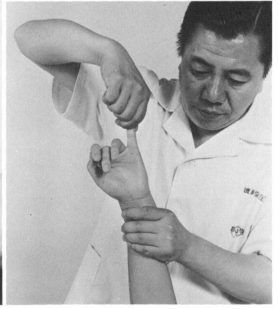

extended straight, the therapist holds her wrist joint in his left hand and, pulling her little-finger tip with his right hand, vibrates the arm (Figs. 7 and 8).

3. Having the patient lie in the prone position, the therapist treats the four points in the right and left supra- and infraorbital regions simultaneously. He applies light palm pressure for ten seconds, two or three times to the eyeballs. This controls pulse by stimulating the Aschner's, or oculocardiac, reflex.

4. The therapist treats the four points on the intercostal areas of the right and left pectoral regions (Fig. 5). Special care is taken to treat the left pectoral region to relax the pectoral and intercostal muscles. Then he treats the sternal body, applies circular palm pressure to the pectoral region, and strokes downward across the pectoral region.

5. In the abdominal region, treatment is concentrated on the epigastric fossa, which must be relaxed thoroughly (Fig. 9).

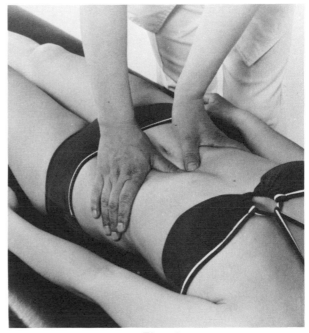

Fig. 9

2. Hypertension (High Blood Pressure)

Maximum blood pressure of more than 160 (when the heart is contracted) and minimum pressure of more than 90 (when the heart is dilated) is considered hypertension, which is of two kinds: essential hypertension, which is unaccompanied by other pathological irregularities and which depends strongly on hereditary elements, and secondary hypertension, which can be caused by the obstructions in the kidneys, the arteries, and the endocrine system, Basedow's disease, or other factors. The term *hypertension*, however, is usually used for essential hypertension.

Persistent hypertension can cause heaviness in the head, dizziness, buzzing in the ears, insomnia, stiffness in the shoulders, constipation, emotional instability, irritability, and excessive excitability. It can lead to cerebral hemorrhage; people who are highly emotional and tense are more liable to this condition than others. Since the brain consumes 20 percent of all the oxygen used by the body, it requires large supplies of blood. When the cerebral blood vessels harden or become brittle, sudden emotional upset causes blood pressure to rise sharply. When this happens, the blood vessels break, resulting in cerebral hemorrhage.

The parts of Japan where rice is the stable food and where large amounts of salty foods are eaten show the highest rates of hypertension. The sodium in salt increases tension in the smooth muscles of the artery walls, causing the arterioles to contract and thus raising blood pressure. Excessive intake of rice brings on accumulation of neutral fats in the body, which, in turn, causes arteriosclerosis. Careful regulation of such foods is essential to the prevention of hypertension.

Hypertension is a serious condition that causes several other pathological complications. By putting a heavy load on it, hypertension causes hypertrophy of the heart and other cardiac ailments. Hardening of the arterioles can bring on renal insufficiency. Consequently, people who have this condition must follow a sensible health program seriously and regularly.

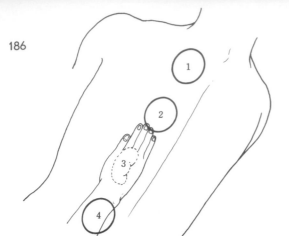

Fig. 10 Pressure Application to the Left
Kidney Region in the Left Lateral Position

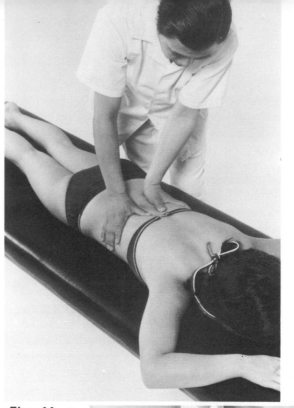

Fig. 11 ▲

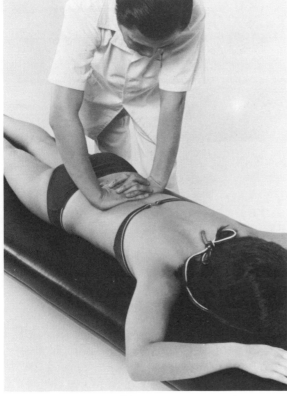

Fig. 14

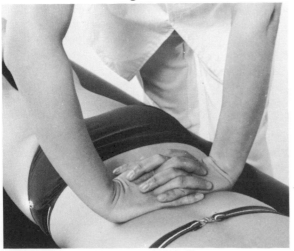

Fig. 13
◄

Fig. 12
►

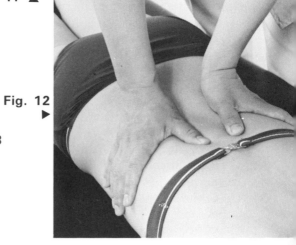

Fig. 15 Extension of the Leg

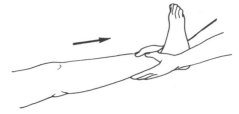

Fig. 16 Extension of the Arm

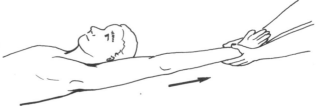

Shiatsu Therapy

General therapy is needed over the entire body, but treatment should be concentrated on the interscapular region (related to the organs of respiration), the infrascapular region (renal area), the extremities of the arms and legs, and the abdomen.

1. Having the patient lie in the left lateral position, the therapist applies light, slow pressure to the entire cervical region, beginning with the anterior cervical region.

2. He then presses five or six times on the five points in the suprascapular and interscapular regions and then on the ten points beginning with the fifth point in the interscapular region and continuing through the infrascapular region into the lumbar region. Next, he applies single-palm pressure for five seconds on each of the four points in Fig. 10 and repeats this therapy five or six times. Finally, he uses vibrational pressure. Palm pressure on the third point in the left renal area is especially important.

3. Having the patient lie in the prone position, the therapist thoroughly treats and relaxes the right and left interscapular regions. Then, with both thumbs, he carefully treats the right and left renal regions simultaneously (Fig. 11). Next, interlocking the fingers of both hands, he presses each point for five seconds with the bases of his hands. He repeats this five or six times (Figs. 13 and 14). Finally, he applies vibrational pressure.

Hypertension can cause sclerosis of the renal arterioles, with a consequent reduction of blood circulation to the kidneys and impairment of their ability to remove liquids and wastes from the body and edema. This treatment is intended to restore the kidneys to normal functioning order.

4. First treating the posterior surfaces of the legs while the patient is still lying in the prone position, the therapist then has the patient assume the supine position so that he can treat the anterior surfaces. After careful therapy on both sides, he finally extends the legs as shown in Fig. 15.

5. With the patient lying in the supine position, the therapist treats the extremities of both arms and then extends the arms (Fig. 16).

6. After lightly treating the head region, he applies slow, gentle palm pressure to the eyeballs.

7. After thorough treatment of the pectoral region, he applies circular palm pressure.

8. After thorough treatment of the entire abdomen, he concentrates on gentle pressure on the epigastric fossa area and the right and left inferior costal regions (Fig. 17). To stimulate digestion and prevent constipation, he carefully treats the sigmoid colon.

9. Finally, once again having the patient assume the prone position, to relax the diaphragm, which tends to tense easily, he performs up-down palm pressure on the right and left lateral abdominal regions (Fig. 18).

Fig. 17 Abdominal Region

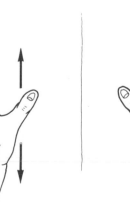

right interior costal region

epigastric fossa

left inferior costal region

sigmoid-colon region

Fig. 18 Up-down Palm Pressure on the Diaphragm in the Prone Position

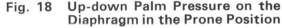
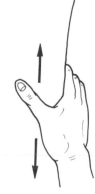

3. Arteriosclerosis

As the human body ages, the arteries sometimes undergo a development leading to a condition known as arteriosclerosis, which is intimately related to cardiac illnesses and hypertension. The highly elastic and contractive arteries are composed of three layers: the adventitia, the media, and the intima and transport blood from the heart to the extremities of the body. Sclerosis may occur in any of the three layers of the arteries. Fat accumulating on the walls of the intima can gradually build up until it narrows the vessel and inhibits the flow of blood. This condition, which is called atherosclerosis (atheroma), occurs readily in large arteries, like the aorta, the coronary arteries, the carotid arteries, the cerebral arteries, and the arteries of the legs.

Hardening of the media occurs in the medium muscular arteries, like the femoral arteries, popliteal arteries, tibial arteries, and radial arteries, when lime depositions form on their walls. This condition is common among elderly people and is found in association with atherosclerosis.

Sclerosis of the adventitia occurs in arterioles. In the brain and kidneys, the adventitia of the arteries hardens and thickens, constricting the inner passage. This condition is related to hypertension.

Though the word *arteriosclerosis* is used in general application, the natures of scleroses vary according to the part of the artery affected and the bodily condition of the individual. Nor is this condition limited to old people. The most important way to prevent arteriorsclerosis is to be constantly aware of your own bodily condition and to follow a sensible health program. Special care should be taken to limit intake of cholesterol. Regularly living habits must be observed; and tobacco, which aggravates arteriosclerosis, should be avoided—best of all, abandoned entirely.

Shiatsu Therapy

1. Having the patient assume the *seiza* kneeling position, the therapist treats the first anterior cervical point, the first lateral cervical point, the medulla-oblongata region, and the

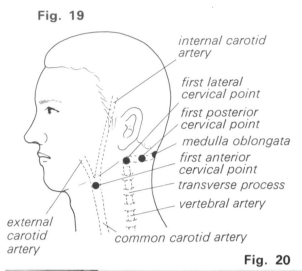

Fig. 19

internal carotid artery
first lateral cervical point
first posterior cervical point
medulla oblongata
first anterior cervical point
transverse process
vertebral artery
external carotid artery
common carotid artery

Fig. 20

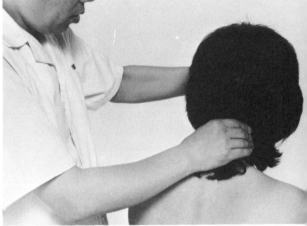

first posterior cervical point in that order (Fig. 19). The posterior cervical point should be especially thoroughly treated to help control obesity (Fig. 20).

2. Having the patient lie in the prone position, the therapist applies pressure with palm and thumb to the renal ergion (Figs. 21 and 22).

3. He then treats the legs and feet in this order: the posterior femoral region, the popliteal fossa, and the plantar region.

4. Next, he treats the arm from the axilla to the cubital fossa, the wrist joint, and the digits.

5. Next, with the patient in the same position, he treats the inguinal region, the anterior femoral region, the anterior crural region, the dorsal surface of the foot, and the digital region. Finally, he treats the abdominal region carefully (Fig. 23).

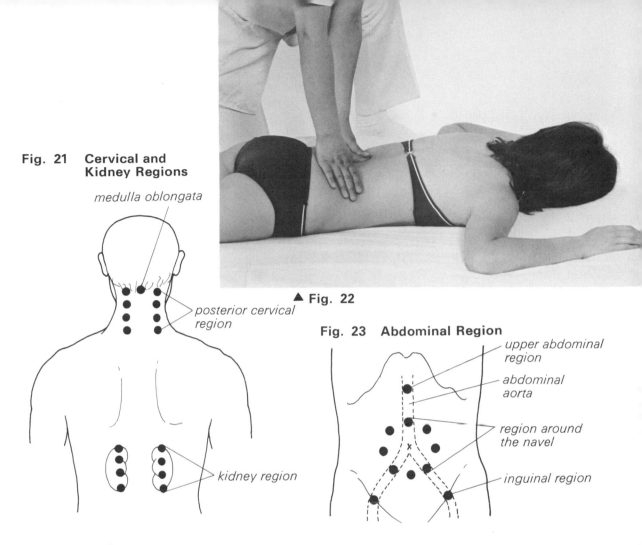

Fig. 21　Cervical and
　　　　Kidney Regions

medulla oblongata

posterior cervical
region

kidney region

▲ Fig. 22

Fig. 23　Abdominal Region

upper abdominal
region

abdominal
aorta

region around
the navel

inguinal region

Neuropathy

1.　Hemiplegia (Paralysis of One Side of the Body)

Hemiplegia is the usual symptom following an attack of cerebral hemorrhage caused by sclerosis of the cerebral blood vessels, which burst under sudden emotional strain. Called convulsive paralysis, this condition manifests itself gradually after the patient regains consciousness from the paroxysm and incapacitates the half of the body opposite to the side on which the cerebral hemorrhage took place. Symptoms appear in the lower part of the face, where paralysis of the muscle groups in the cheeks, nose, and mouth hinders speech. Owing to contracture of the pectoral muscle, the arm is turned inward against the trunk (adduction). The antebrachial region, wrist joint, and digits are bent

as if in contraction (flexion and pronation). The hip joint is twisted outward (abduction), and the crural region hangs flaccid and overextended. The foot is turned in (talipes varus), and the digits are extended and cause talipes equinus. This syndrome of symptoms is called Wernicke-Mann type contracture (Fig. 24). Talipes equinus causes the patient to swing the afflicted foot in an arc as he walks. It is extremely difficult to restore to normal walking ability a person suffering from a serious case of Wernicke-Mann type contracture. But, as soon as possible after the patient regains consciousness, the following therapy should be performed, under the guidance of a physician.

Shiatsu Therapy

1. Having the patient lie in the supine position, the therapist first slowly treats the pectoralis major muscle, the deltopectoral groove, and the deltoid muscle (Fig. 25) to prevent adduction of the shoulder joint (Fig. 26).

2. He applies continuous pressure with a pull in the direction of the fingers on the arm in this order: triceps brachii, anconeus muscle, supinator muscle, the group of extensor muscles, the wrist joint, and the interdigital joints to the ends of the fingers (Figs. 27 and 28).

3. To prevent abduction of the hip joint, the therapist carefully treats and relaxes the group of adductor muscles in the medial femoral region.

4. Having the patient assume the prone position, the therapist treats the flexor muscle in the posterior femoral region to prevent hyperextension of the knee joint (Fig. 30).

5. Having the patient return to the supine position, the therapist relaxes the anterior tibial muscle and the fibularis muscle group to prevent plantarflexion and talipes verus. He puts the foot through dorsiflextion exercises to extend the muscles in the plantar region and thus to prevent talipes equinus (Fig. 31). Plantarflexion to exercise the opposition muscles must not be forgotten.

6. He performs thorough treatment on the abdomen to prevent constipation, which often accompanies this condition (Fig. 33).

When this treatment is completed, the patient should be guided in using the hand and fingers of the sound side to conduct self-administered shiatsu on the afflicted side and to move those parts of the body unaided. Finally, to prevent contracture during sleep, the afflicted limbs should be wrapped with towels or pieces of blanket.

Hemiplegia patients who lie in bed a long time

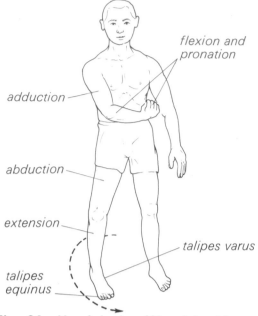

Fig. 24 Hemiplegia—Wernicke-Mann-type Contracture

are subject to decubitus especially at the sacrum, greater trochanter, ilium, spinous processes of the vertebrae, and scapulae. Because muscular contraction removes fat from the body, the action of sweat and wrinkles in bedding tend to cause inflamation of the patient's skin in these regions. To prevent this condition sweat should be wiped dry as soon as possible; and bedding should be smoothed from time to time. The patient's body should be moved during this process.

Fig. 26

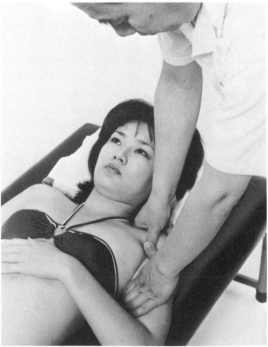

Fig. 25 Deltoid Muscle, Deltopectoral Groove, and Pectoral Region

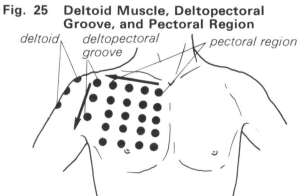

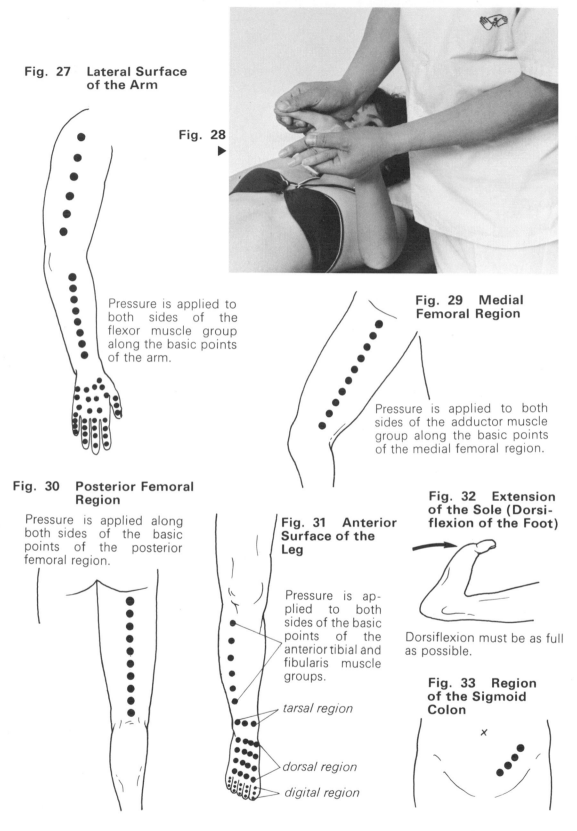

Fig. 27   Lateral Surface of the Arm

Fig. 28

Pressure is applied to both sides of the flexor muscle group along the basic points of the arm.

Fig. 29   Medial Femoral Region

Pressure is applied to both sides of the adductor muscle group along the basic points of the medial femoral region.

Fig. 30   Posterior Femoral Region

Pressure is applied along both sides of the basic points of the posterior femoral region.

Fig. 31   Anterior Surface of the Leg

Pressure is applied to both sides of the basic points of the anterior tibial and fibularis muscle groups.

tarsal region

dorsal region

digital region

Fig. 32   Extension of the Sole (Dorsi-flexion of the Foot)

Dorsiflexion must be as full as possible.

Fig. 33   Region of the Sigmoid Colon

2. Insomnia

Some of the causes of prolonged inability to sleep are worry and stress, encephalemia, neural hypersensitivity, and arteriosclerosis. Sometimes worry about inability to sleep aggravates the condition, but this is no reason to become reliant on sleeping drugs.

Fig. 34

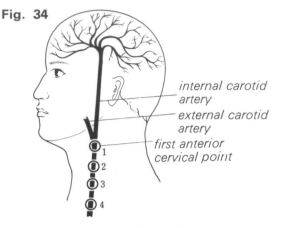

internal carotid artery

external carotid artery

first anterior cervical point

Fig. 35

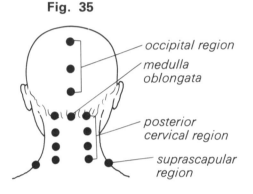

occipital region

medulla oblongata

posterior cervical region

suprascapular region

Fig. 36

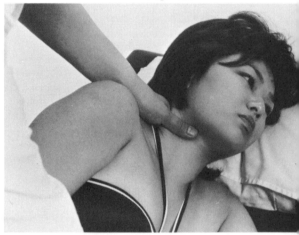

Fig. 37

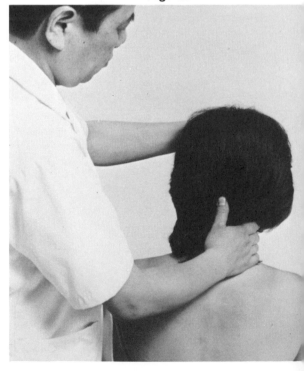

Shiatsu Therapy
People who suffer from insomnia are stiff in the abdomen and cervical region. Treatment must be concentrated in these areas.

1.   Having the patient kneel in the *seiza* position, the therapist treats the first point in the anterior cervical region (Fig. 34) and then goes on to treat the anterior cervical region, lateral cervical region, medulla-oblongata region, and posterior cervical region (Figs. 36 and 37). This stimulates transport of fresh blood to the brain by means of the common carotid artery, internal carotid artery, and vertebral arteries and thus speeds the return of waste blood by way of the veins.

2.   Careful treatment is applied to the occipital region, the suprascapular region, the dorsal region, and all parts of the legs and arms. Then the six points on the median line of the head are treated, with sustained, then vibrational pressure on the sixth point (Fig. 38). Palm pressure is applied to the eyeballs—ten seconds per point.

3.   Pressure is then applied to soften the abdomen in the vicinity of the diaphragm.

Fig. 38

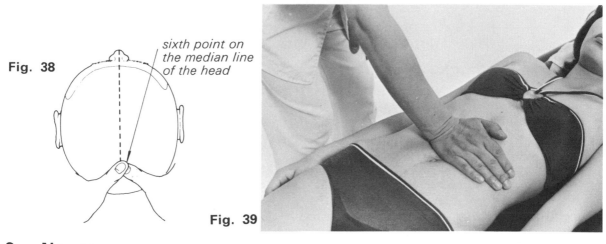

sixth point on the median line of the head

Fig. 39

3. Neuroses

Nervous reactions and neurasthenia, manifesting themselves in mental instability, moodiness, inability to concentrate, abnormality in speech and actions, and many other pathological symptoms, affect people of all ages. They are brought on by psychological elements like domestic upsets, trouble in human relations, hardships related to work, shocks suffered in childhood, and so on. People who are of weak psychological constitution, who fret, and who become hysterical easily are prone to neuroses. But conditions of this kind, unlike such graver mental illnesses as manic-depressive psychosis, can be cured through the patient's own mental attitude and through the understanding and guidance of the people around them.

Shiatsu Therapy
The full course of shiatsu therapy—with special attention to the total cervical region, occipital region, medulla-oblongata region, suprascapular region, back, and head (especially the sixth point on the median line) should be carried out. To it should be added palm pressure on the temporal region and the eyeballs. Finally, the diaphragm region should be thoroughly limbered (Figs. 40 through 43), since this stimulates digestion. It is very important to prevent indigestion, constipation, and diarrhea. In addition, the patient should get plenty of sleep and remain calm.

Fig. 40 Palm Pressure on Six Points of the Median Line of the Temporal Region

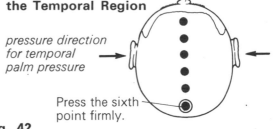

pressure direction for temporal palm pressure

Press the sixth point firmly.

Fig. 41

Fig. 42

Fig. 43 Epigastric Fossa and Palm Pressure on the Eyeballs

palm pressure on the eyeballs

epigastric fossa

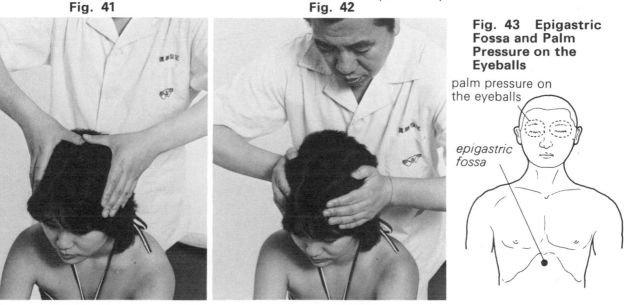

4. Trigeminal Neuralgia

Trigeminal neuralgia is of two types: idiopathic trigeminal neuralgia, the causes of which are uncertain; and symptomatic trigeminal neuralgia caused by aneurysma, sinus disease, gingivitis, and metabolic abnormalities.

The thickest of the cranial nerves, the trigeminal (three-branched) nerve arises in the fifth cranial nerve and forms the semilunar ganglion (Gasserian's ganglion) and then branches into three parts. The first branch is the ophthalmic nerve, the second is the maxillary nerve, and the third, the mandibular nerve. These nerves are distributed all over the face (Fig. 44). Pain-pressure points for the three branches differ; that for the first branch is at the supraorbital foramen; that for the second branch, at the infraorbital foramen and the zygomaticofacial foramen; and that for the third branch at the mental foramen (Fig. 45). But pain almost never occurs in more than one of these nerves at the same time. In the case of the first branch, pain occurs at the root of the nose, the supraorbital region, and the frontal region. In the case of the second branch, it occurs in the infraorbital region, the area of the zygomatic bone, the wings of the nose, and the upper lip. In the case of the third branch, it occurs in the mandible, the lower lip, the vicinity of the ears, and the temporal region.

Shiatsu Therapy

Centering treatment on the pressure-pain points, the therapist uses fluid pressure, sustained pressure, vibrational pressure, and pressure relaxed then reapplied in accordance with the demands of the symptoms (Fig. 46). When pain is caused by the first branch of the trigeminal nerve, thumb, three-finger, or palm pressure should be used on the four points in the supraorbital region. Then the thumb or three fingers are used to treat the points on the outside of the median line in the frontal region (Fig. 47). When pain is caused by the second branch, the therapist uses thumbs or three fingers to treat the four points in the infraorbital region, the three points in the zygomatic region from the side of the nose to the ear, and the three points on the upper lip from the inside outward (Fig. 48). When pain is caused by the third branch of the trigeminal nerve, treatment is performed on the three mandibular points and on the gums in this area (Fig. 49) with either the thumbs or three fingers. Then, since moving the mouth in cases of this kind of complaint is painful, the oral area too is treated with light pressure.

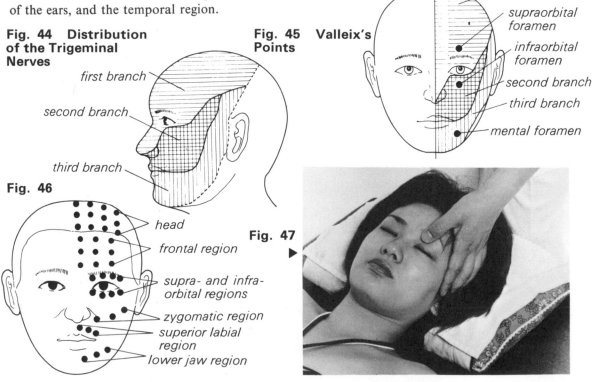

Fig. 44 Distribution of the Trigeminal Nerves

first branch

second branch

third branch

Fig. 45 Valleix's Points

first branch

supraorbital foramen

infraorbital foramen

second branch

third branch

mental foramen

Fig. 46

head

frontal region

supra- and infra-orbital regions

zygomatic region

superior labial region

lower jaw region

Fig. 47

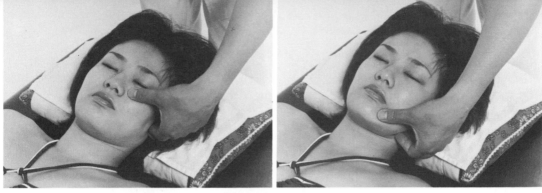

Fig. 48   Fig. 49

5. Occipital Neuralgia

Occipital neuralgia occurs in the region where the major occipital nerve, minor occipital nerve, third occipital nerve, and great auricular nerve are distributed and from the nuchal region through the top part of the occipital zone in one or both lateral regions. Valleix's point appears either between the mastoid process and the first cervical vertebra or between the mastoid process and the medulla oblongata (Fig. 50). The cause of the trouble may be induration of the muscles and adipose tissues in the occipital region, tension in the nuchal ligament, arteriosclerosis, or the so-called whiplash-syndrome.

Shiatsu Therapy

1. The therapist relaxes tension in the occipital region by repeated thumb-on-thumb pressure on the three points between the mastoid process and the medulla oblongata on the afflicted side (Fig. 51). The second point is the location of the tender point and therefore requires especially careful treatment (Fig. 52).

2. Using the three points between the mastoid process and the medulla oblongata as the starters, the therapist treats three vertical rows of points—four over and including the first in the horizontal row, five over and including the second in the horizontal row, and six over and including the third in the horizontal row—(Fig. 51) in the order stated, from bottom upward.

3. Turning the afflicted side of the patient's face slightly outward, the therapist places the palm of one hand against the bottom of the occipital bone (inferior nuchal border) and the opposite hand against the patient's forehead and extends the entire occipital region upward for five seconds (Fig. 53). This is repeated three times. Then, with the base of the hand on the occipital region, he applies vibrational pressure about three times. When occipital neuralgia

Fig. 50

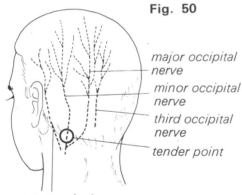

major occipital nerve

minor occipital nerve

third occipital nerve

tender point

great auricular nerve

Fig. 52

Fig. 53

Fig. 51

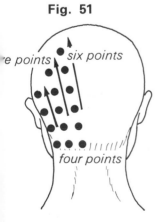

e points   six points

four points

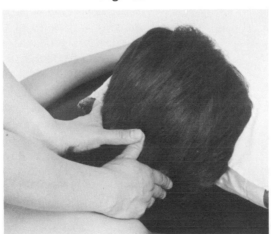

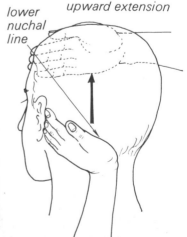

lower nuchal line   upward extension

occurs in both lateral zones simultaneously, the therapist begins on the left and then repeats the same therapy on the right.

4. Thorough shiatsu must be applied to the lateral cervical, medulla-oblongata, and occipital regions.

6. Brachial Neuralgia

Localized pain occurs in the arms according to the distribution of the brachial nerves. For instance, the axillary nerve causes pain in the deltoid muscle and the teres minor muscle (movement of the brachial region); the musculocutaneous nerve causes pain in the biceps brachii muscle, the coracobrachial muscle, the brachial muscle (movement of the antebrachial region); the ulnar nerve, the median nerve, and the radial nerve cause pain in the antebrachial region, the carpus, the dorsal region of the hand, the palmar region of the hand, and the phalangeal joints (Fig. 54).

Shiatsu Therapy

The therapist must perform sustained treatment on the afflicted zones, centering treatment on the courses of the nerves. He must extend the shoulder joint, the elbow joint, the wrist joint, and the interphalangeal joints (Fig. 55). In this extremely important extending technique, he must work gradually and slowly to extend the nerves.

Fig. 55

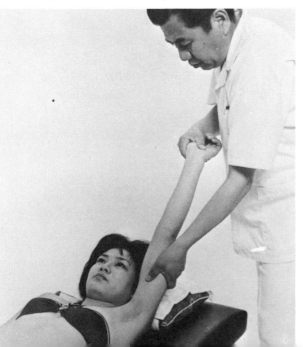

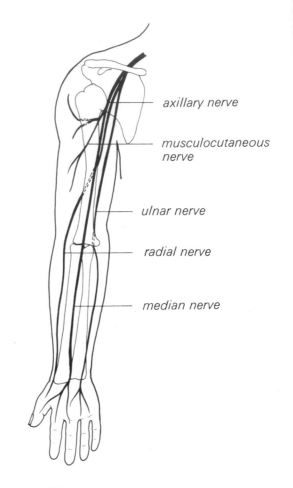

axillary nerve

musculocutaneous nerve

ulnar nerve

radial nerve

median nerve

Fig. 54 Anterior Surface of the Right Arm

7. Intercostal Neuralgia

The intercostal nerves arising from the right and left sides of the vertebrae pass downward diagonally across the lateral abdominal region in the intercostal zone and then diagonally upward to both sides of the sternal body. Intercostal neuralgia, generally affecting only one side, is most common in the left lateral region, especially in the fifth through the ninth intercostal nerves. Pain is usually in bands in the pectoral, dorsal, and lateral abdominal regions and may be accompanied by herpes. It occurs often on the left side and is frequently referred to as a cutaneovisceral reflex. Though actual respiration is unaffected, breathing causes pain.

There are three Valleix's points: vertebral, lateral pectoral, and sternal (Fig. 56). All three of them are placed where cutaneous nerves are located.

Causes for intercostal neuralgia include rigidity of the erector spinae muscles and the intercostal muscles, heart ailments, and irregularities in the vertebral column or the ribs.

Shiatsu Therapy

When pain is in the frontal pectoral region, the patient assumes the lateral position; and the therapist treats the interscapular and infrascapular regions. Then, having the patient lie supine, he gently presses the afflicted side from the sternal body to the ribs (Fig. 57). Thumb pressure, three-finger pressure, and palm pressure are used.

When the pain is in the dorsal or lateral abdominal regions, all treatment is performed with the patient lying on her side. In this case, the therapist assumes a position beside the patient's head and, raising her arm above her head, treats the lateral abdominal region (Fig. 58). Thumb pressure, three-finger pressure, palm pressure, and vibrational pressure are used. In both instances, the therapist must devote special attention to treating the diaphragm and must have the patient breathe deeply and quietly while he attempts to relieve the pain.

Fig. 56   Tender Points in Intercostal Neuralgia

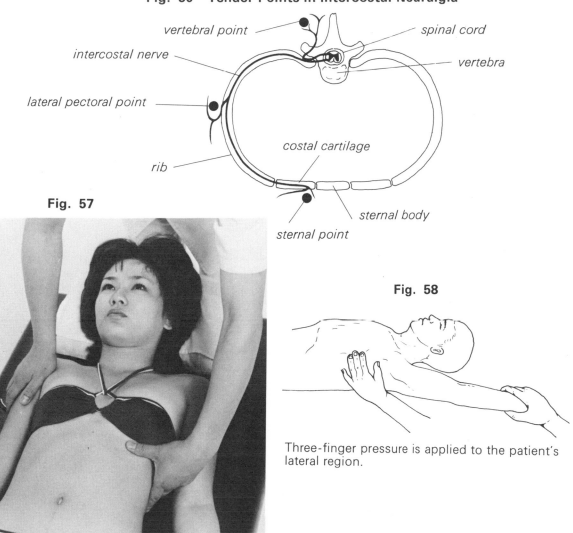

Fig. 57

Fig. 58

Three-finger pressure is applied to the patient's lateral region.

8. Sciatica

The roots of the sciatic nerve are in the fourth and fifth lumbar and the first, second, and third sacral vertebrae. Extending from this place, where they are in a bundle, they pass through the posterior femoral and posterior crural regions and to the plantar region and the digits of the feet. They are the longest and thickest —the thickness of the little digit—peripheral nerves in the body. Most often sciatica results from hernias in the intervertebral discs. But other causes include deformations of the vertebrae, irregularities in the sacroiliac joint, hypertrophy of the flaval ligament attached to the posterior vertebral foramen, and rigidity in the surrounding ligaments and muscles.

The tender point is between the sciatic tuber and the greater trochanter on the afflicted side. If this condition becomes chronic, attempts to ease the pain cause people to lean in the direction of the sound side in a condition called sciatic scoliosis.

Lasègue's sign is a famous method of diagnosing sciatica. The patient is made to lie supine. The therapist raises the entire leg without allowing the patient to bend the knee joint (Fig. 60). In people suffering from sciatica, this causes sharp pain in the sciatic nerve in the posterior femoral region. Bending the foot intensifies the pain.

Shiatsu Therapy
First, having the patient lie prone, the therapist thoroughly treats the lumbar region, gluteal region, and Namikoshi point, in this order. Next he uses sustained pressure on the Valleix's points along the course of the sciatic nerve (Fig. 59). Then he treats the entire leg, with special attention to the posterior side.

Next, having the patient assume the supine position, he carefully and slowly treats the abdominal region—especially the lower abdomen—to relieve chilling and stiffness and to prevent constipation. Since the sciatic nerve is relatively close to the surface of the skin, care must be taken not to sit long in damp or cold places and to keep the afflicted part of the body warm at all times.

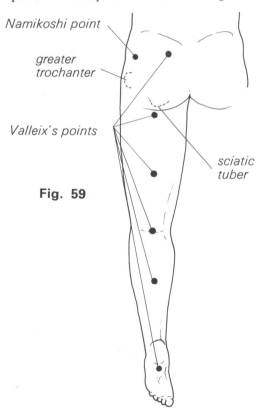

Namikoshi point

greater trochanter

Valleix's points

sciatic tuber

Fig. 59

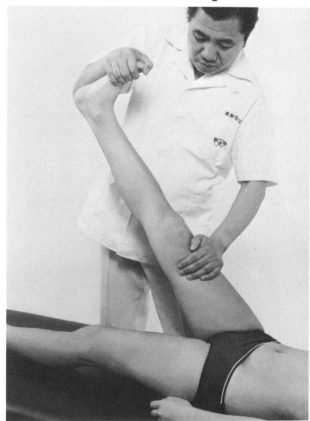

Fig. 60

Fig. 61 An Instance of Alopecia Areata

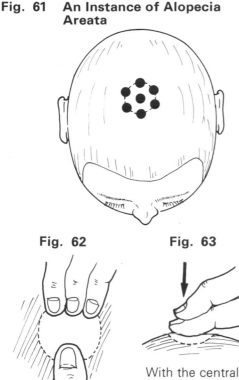

Fig. 62   **Fig. 63**

With the central part as support, pressure is applied with the index and middle fingers.

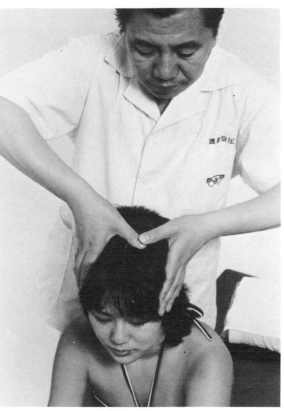

Fig. 64

9. Alopecia Areata

Alopecia areata, or sudden balding in patches, occurs because of obstructions of circulation to the scalp and resultant lack of sufficient nutrition to the hair roots. It is not contagious; and, since it is accompanied by neither itching nor pain, it often is cured before the afflicted person is aware that he has the condition. It sometimes occurs in more than one place at the same time.

Psychological causes are frequently behind the condition, which develops in people who are worried, are excited, suffer from accumulated stress, or are subject to extreme tension over long periods. Migraine and insomnia are sometimes the cause.

Shiatsu Therapy

1. After having the patient wash her hair, the therapist uses either thumbs or three fingers—index, middle, and ring—to press the center and the periphery of the balding patch carefully (Figs. 61 and 62).

2. Then he applies vibrational thumb-on-thumb presssure to the center of the patch (Fig. 63). He next uses thumb-on-thumb pressure to treat the median line, both temporal regions, the parietal zone, and the medulla-oblongata region (Fig. 64).

3. Next he presses the cervical and supra-scapular regions, which are often stiff in cases of this condition.

4. He further treats the abdominal region to stimulate good digestion and ensure ample nutrition to the hair roots.

Fig. 65 Frontal, Orbital, and Temple Regions

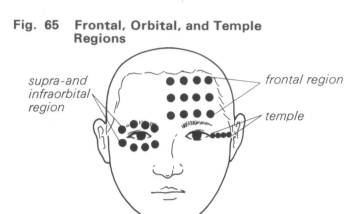

supra-and infraorbital region

frontal region

temple

Fig. 66 Temporal Region

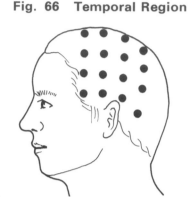

Fig. 67 Occipital Region

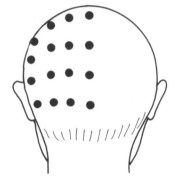

Fig. 68

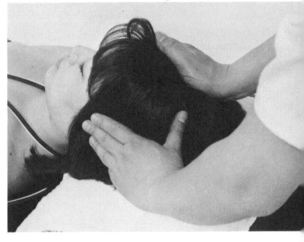

10. Migraine

This kind of headache, which most often afflicts women, occurs in only parts of the head, for example the temporal, frontal, or occipital regions or behind the eyes, and is accompanied by such preliminary symptoms as nausea, dizziness, buzzing in the ears, and flashing spots in front of the eyes. Related to the blood vessels, migraine frequently occurs when the person has eaten something stimulating that causes the vessels to expand. It occurs in high-blood-pressure patients, insomniacs, and people who have hardened muscles that cause contraction of the blood vessels.

Shiatsu Therapy

1. The therapist begins by holding the unafflicted side of the head of the patient, who is in the *seiza* kneeling position, in one hand and applying palm pressure to the afflicted part with the other hand for five to ten seconds. The degree of pressure must be gauged to the severity of the symptoms. Vibrational pressure too may be used.

2. Other points for pressure depend on the location of the pain. In the case of frontal pain, there are four vertical rows of points leading from the median frontal line across the forehead above the eyebrows. For pain in the orbital region, there are four points in the supraorbital region, four in the infraorbital region and an additional four in the temples (Fig. 65). For pain in the temporal region, there are four rows of points leading from the median line to the temporal region on the afflicted side (Fig. 66). For pain in the occipital region, there are four rows of four points from the median line to the affected side of the occipital region. All of these points must be treated (Fig. 68).

3. Then, without special attention to the location of the pain, the therapist treats the entire cervical region.

11. Subacute Myelo-optico-neuropathy (SMON Disease)

This sickness, which occurred in large numbers of people all over Japan between 1968 and 1970 and caused intense suffering and concern, was discovered to have been caused by an intestinal medicine called chinoform. When this was ascertained, in September 1970, production of the medicine was outlawed; and, since that time, no new cases have developed. In the early stages of the illness the patient complains of diarrhea and abdominal pains. Then sensory stimuli—prickly sensations like those caused by walking barefoot on sand—appear in the extremities of the feet. Reflexes in the Achilles' tendon weaken and then fail entirely. This condition advances to hypersensitive reactions in the patellar reflex and

to positive Babinski's signs (see p. 30). Numbness, pain, and abnormal sensations progress gradually upward from the legs to the navel and the chest. In serious cases, motion of the legs becomes impossible; and numbness, pain, and disability advance as far as the arms.

Shiatsu Therapy
The therapist must conduct total-body treatment lasting for no more than forty or fifty minutes: longer than this may tire the patient and have adverse effects on the treatment.

Special attention must be devoted to sustained and vibrational pressure on the occipital region, medulla-oblongata region, anterior cervical region, suprascapular region, and both sides of the vertebral column through the interscapular region to the lumbar region and the Namikoshi point (Fig. 69). He should then devote careful treatment to the arms and legs, especially the crural region and the first point in the lateral antebrachial region (Fig. 70). Depending on the symptoms, light pressure, standard pressure, interrupted pressure, and sustained pressure should be applied to other parts.

He must use sustained pressure in areas where the skin is chilled in order to stimulate cutaneous functioning and thus prevent stiffness and roughness. This will in turn stimulate circulation in the capillaries and relieve pain.

Finally, thorough palm pressure must be given to the abdominal region (Figs. 71 and 72) to restore good functioning in the stomach and intestines, stimulate digestion, improve assimilation of nutrients, and prevent diarrhea and constipation.

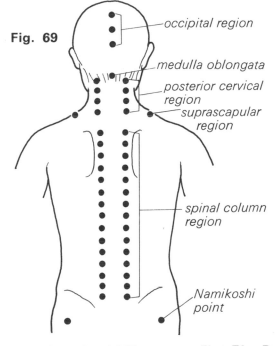

Fig. 69

occipital region
medulla oblongata
posterior cervical region
suprascapular region
spinal column region
Namikoshi point

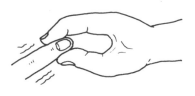

Fig. 70 Sustained Vibrational Pressure for the Extremities of the Arms and Legs

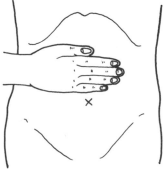

Fig. 71 Palm Pressure on the Abdominal Region

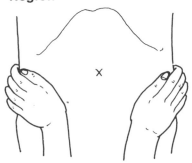

Fig. 72 Palm Pressure on the Lateral Abdominal Region

Ailments in the Alimentary Organs

1. Diarrhea

Weakening of the functioning of the stomach and intestines or chilling in the legs and lumbar region causes poor digestion. Materials left undigested stimulate the mucous membrane of the colon and accelerate peristalsis with the result that the contents pass rapidly through the tract before liquid is adequately absorbed and the contents reach the rectum in a semifluid state. This causes diarrhetic defecation. Sometimes imbalance in the autonomic nerves excites the parasympathetic nerves, causing accelerated passage of partly digested materials through the colon.

Persistent diarrhea dehydrates the body and prevents assimilation of nutrients, thus lowering resistance power and producing a state of debility. To prevent this, it is a good idea to use shiatsu therapy to stimulate digestion and to regulate the operation of the intestines. Virus-caused colds frequently bring on attacks of diarrhea, especially in children. It is therefore advisable to use shiatsu treatment to maintain good health and resistance against colds. In addition, shiatsu is effective in restoring general good health.

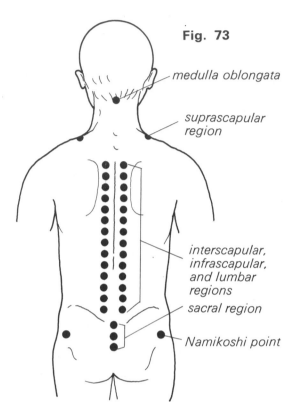

Fig. 73

medulla oblongata

suprascapular region

interscapular, infrascapular, and lumbar regions

sacral region

Namikoshi point

Fig. 74

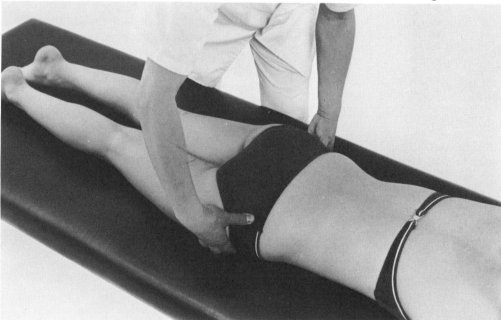

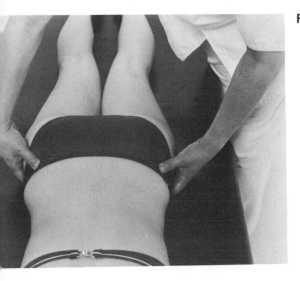

Fig. 75   Fig. 76   Fig. 77

first dorsal point (between
the roots of the first and
second toes)

six points in the
lateral crural
region

Fig. 78

Shiatsu Therapy

1. Having the patient lie prone, the therapist treats the medulla-oblongata region, the right and left surpascapular regions, the interscapular region, the infrascapular region, the lumbar region, and the sacral region (Fig. 73) to regulate the autonomic nervous system and control excessive peristalsis in the intestines.

2. Then he simultaneously applies thumb pressure to both Namikoshi points (Figs. 74 and 75), five seconds per point, with treatment repeated from three to five times.

3. Then, having the patient lie supine, he applies pressure to the six points in the lateral crural region from the patellar joint to a point just above the ankle joint. Treatment lasts for five seconds on each point and is repeated from three to five times.

4. Next, strong pressure is used on the ankle joint and the dorsal surface of the foot, with special attention being paid to the fossae between the bases of the first and second digits (Fig. 77). To stimulate circulation in the legs, treatment is given to the digits and to the plantar surface of the foot.

5. Palm pressure is applied simultaneously to the left and right lateral abdominal regions (Fig. 78). After this is repeated three times, palm pressure is applied for five seconds to each of the nine points around the abdomen. This treatment is repeated from three to five times (Fig. 79).

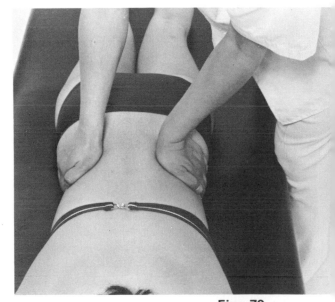

Fig. 79

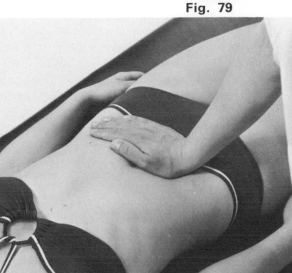

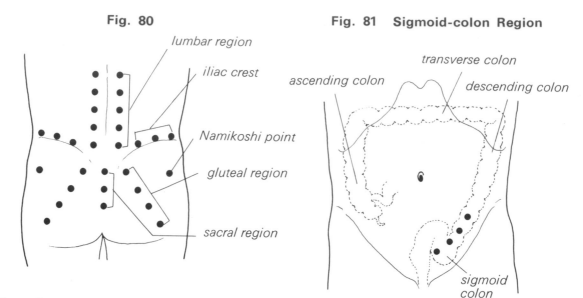

Fig. 80

lumbar region

iliac crest

Namikoshi point

gluteal region

sacral region

Fig. 81 Sigmoid-colon Region

transverse colon

ascending colon

descending colon

sigmoid colon

2. Constipation

Normally defecation occurs once daily. When it is no more frequent than once in three days or once a week, discomfort and the condition called chronic constipation sets in. Often this is caused by upsets in the autonomic nervous system brought on by irregular eating habits or psychological stress. The sympathetic nerves suppress the activity of the alimentary canal, and the parasympathetic nerves stimulate it. When the autonomic nervous system is upset, the action of the parasympathetic nerves is dulled, the functioning of the intestines is repressed, and constipation results. Structurally, the intestines consist of repeated bulging and constricted zones, which alternately relax and contract, setting up the peristaltic motion that is characteristic of them.

Consuming only easily digested foods like bread, cheese, butter, and yogurt out of worry about constipation is unadvisable since, failing to stimulate the colon, such a diet does not activate intestinal peristalsis. Instead of these foods, it is better to eat suitable amounts of vegetables and fruits with cellulose content, which regulates intestinal movement. But, eaten in excessive quantities, these foods too can have an undesirable effect on constipation. Foods like the Japanese salted, dried plum called *umeboshi*; oranges; orange juice; peaches; and avocados,

which contain suitable amounts of both cellulose and organic acids, stimulate the colon and have a regulating effect. Avoiding prolonged use of laxatives, which can be harmful, and patiently carrying out the shiatsu therapy described below regulate the operation of the autonomic nervous system and improve digestive ability.

Shiatsu Therapy

1. First, the therapist treats the anterior cervical region, the region of the medulla oblongata, and the sacral region to stimulate the operation of the parasympathetic nerves.

2. Next, he applies pressure to the lumbar region, the iliac crest, the sacral region, the gluteal region, and the Namikoshi point (Fig. 80). The Namikoshi point has stimulating effects on the intestines.

3. He then treats the entire abdominal region with special emphasis on the nine points located in these places in this order: stomach, small intestine, large intestine, ascending colon, transverse colon, descending colon, sigmoid colon, and rectum. Firm pressure with the thenar must be especially carefully applied to the sigmoid colon (Figs. 81 through 84).

4. Finally fluid and circular palm pressures are applied to the abdomen.

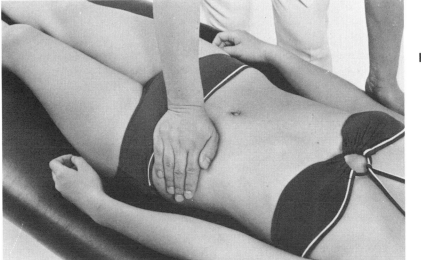

Fig. 82

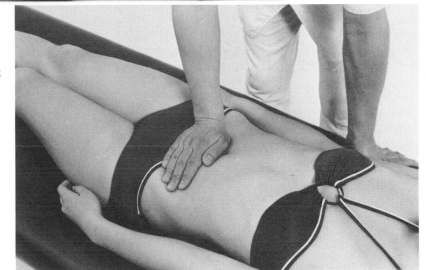

Fig. 83

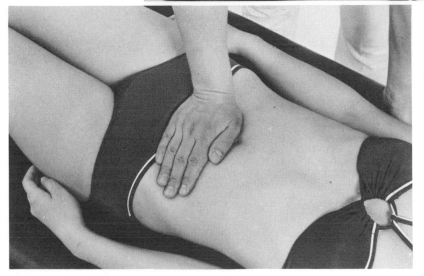

Fig. 84

3. Gastroptosis

For constitutional reasons or as a result of overall debility from pathological causes, the muscular tissues of the stomach can become atonic. If this continues for a long time, maintenance of muscular tonus becomes impossible; and the stomach drops below its normal position above the navel. It slowly falls from a line connecting the left and right iliac crests as far as the pelvic cavity. When this happens, a condition known as gastroptosis, in which the patient suffers from upset stomach, indigestion, belching, and other subjective symptoms, sets in. If these symptoms do not manifest themselves, there is no cause to become nervous about the situation.

Often slender women whose stomach are not especially strong fall victim to this condition and to gastroatony. Such people should follow a regular course of shiatsu therapy to develop muscular strength to maintain tension in the abdominal walls and gradually to improve digestive abilities.

Shiatsu Therapy

1. People prone to gastroptosis tend to be nervous and to suffer from stiffness in the cervical, scapular, and dorsal regions. Treatment should be concentrated on limbering the cervical region and the right and left—especially the left—suprascapular regions.

2. The therapist first treats the area from the interscapular region to the lumbar region on the left side of the vertebral column and then the areas from the interscapular to the lumbar region on the right side of the vertebral column.

3. He then treats the legs carefully all the way to the terminations of the digits to stimulate circulation. It is important to prevent chilling in the lower abdominal region.

4. Having the patient lie prone, the therapist first treats the entire abdomen and then applies circular palm pressure on the stomach region with a suction effect in the direction of the diaphragm (Figs. 85 through 88). It is important to keep the palm of the hand pressed well against

Fig. 85 Circular Rotational Palm Pressure

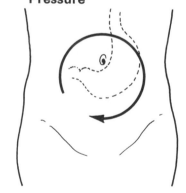

Fig. 86 Suction Pressure

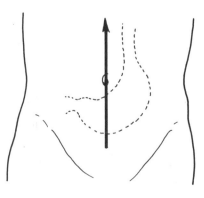

Fig. 87

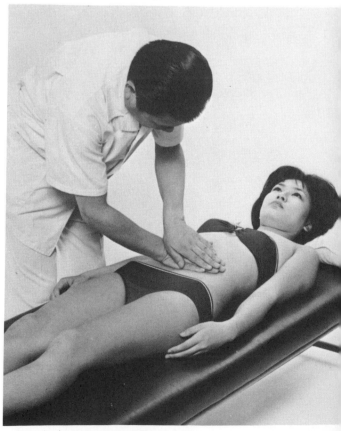

Fig. 88

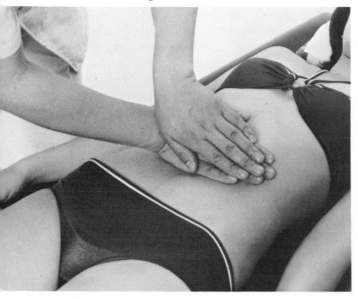

Fig. 89   Suction Pressure

The palm is held firmly against the patient's skin.

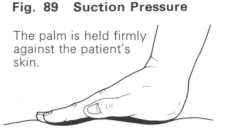

Fig. 90   Upward Kneading on the Abdominal Region

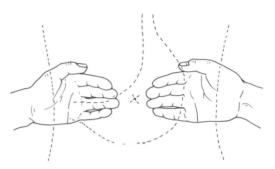

the patient's skin at this time (Fig. 89). This operation, which lasts five seconds, is repeated from five to ten times. Then, slipping his hands under the patient's body slightly lower than normal stomach position and to the sides of the navel, with the digital balls of the four fingers of each hand placed to the right and left side of the patient's vertebral column, the therapist exerts a kneading, upward pressure ten times (Fig. 90).

5.   Finally, the therapist holds the patient's ankle joints and has the patient perform ten sit-ups (Fig. 91). The exercise is more effective if the hands are locked behind the head, but if this is difficult it can be performed with arms extended forward (Fig. 92).

Fig. 91   Exercise A with the Trunk Raised

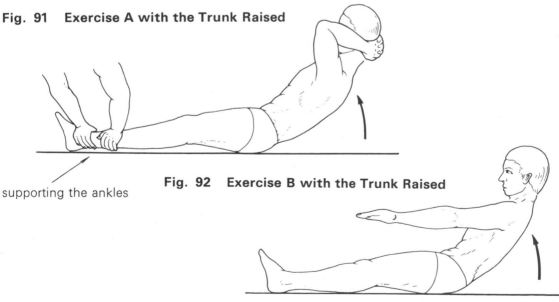

supporting the ankles

Fig. 92   Exercise B with the Trunk Raised

4. Ailments of the Liver

The liver is important to such vital functions as metabolism, evacuation, detoxification, blood production, circulation, and bile secretion. Among the largest of the body organs, it is comparable in size to the brain, weighing from 1,200 to 1,500 grams. The hepatic arteries and the portal veins, which have special, large vessel structures, empty into the liver. The hepatic arteries transport oxygen and nutrients to nourish the liver; and the portal veins transport metabolic products from the stomach, intestines, pancreas, and spleen. In other words, the liver is a storehouse and source of the energy-producing elements abundantly contained in blood.

Major hepatic ailments include hepatitis, hepatocirrhosis, and fatty liver. These conditions, which are caused by overindulgence in food and drink and by accumulated fatigue, often continued to grow more serious without manifesting subjective symptoms. To treat them, it is important to eat appropriate quantities of the right kinds of foods, to avoid accumulated fatigue, and to get ample rest. As the English term for an irascible person *hot liver* suggests, pathological conditions in the liver are often the results of psychological factors. People who tend to be subject to these conditions must avoid irritation and excitement.

Shiatsu Therapy

1. Covered by the ribs, the liver is located immediately below the diaphragm in the upper right abdominal (right infracostal) region (Fig. 93). Ailments in the liver cause a feeling of heavy oppressiveness and dull pain in this region. Tactile investigation there reveals the condition of the liver. Since this is an easy place for self-shiatsu, the individual can readily keep an eye on his own liver condition and regulate it with shiatsu therapy.

First, with both palms—right hand on the bottom—on the lower right costal region, the therapist applies slow, upward, kneading pressure (Fig. 94). If this pressure results in no pain and no feeling of oppressiveness, the liver is in normal condition. Since the liver is large, it is necessary to employ similar tactile investigations

Fig. 93

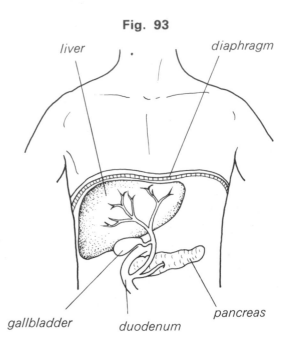

liver   diaphragm

gallbladder   duodenum   pancreas

Fig. 94 Pressure Direction for the Right Inferior Costal (Liver) Region (arrow)

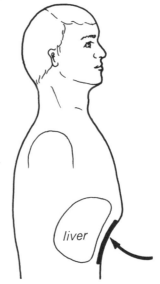

liver

in the area of the diaphragm and in the lateral abdominal region (Fig. 95) to obtain a full understanding of its condition.

2. If this tactile examination of the right lower costal region reveals hardness, first of all, palm pressure and then slight, vibrational pressure (Fig. 96) must be applied there. When the

hardness is limbered, slow thumb pressure should be applied. The same operation is repeated with the index, middle, and ring fingers of one hand. The three fingers must be held together.

3. Then the therapist treats the right suprascapular, interscapular, and infrascapular regions (Fig. 97), while investigating liver functions (Fig. 98). With the exception of treatment of the right interscapular region, this therapy can be self-administered. Performed lightly, daily during the bath or before retiring, it keeps the liver in good condition.

Fig. 95

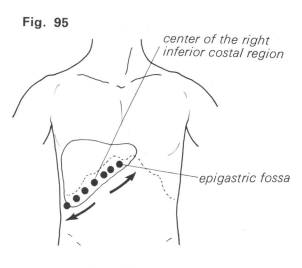

center of the right inferior costal region

epigastric fossa

Fig. 96

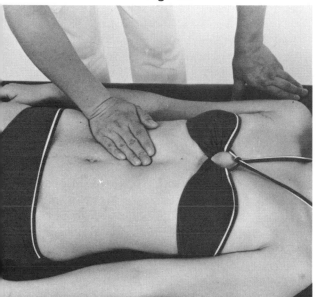

Fig. 97

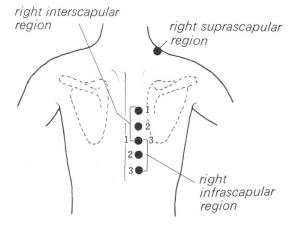

right interscapular region

right suprascapular region

right infrascapular region

Fig. 98

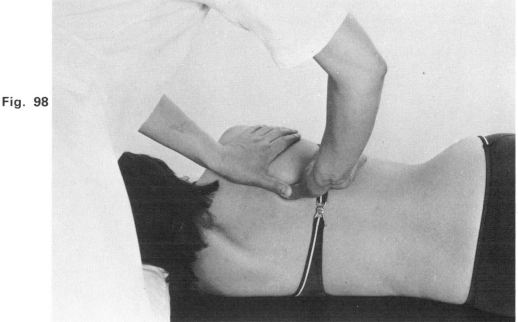

5. Cholelithiasis (Gallstone)

The gallbladder, which is shaped like a small eggplant and is approximately eight centimeters long and four centimeters wide, is attached to the under aspect of the liver. Bile produced in the liver passes through the hepatic duct and the cystic duct to enter the gallbladder, where it is concentrated as a result of absorption of water by means of the bladder walls. Bile is stored in the gallbladder until needed in the digestion of fats and proteins, when it is secreted. The gallbladder contracts as the opening of the duodenum relaxes as a consequence of Oddi's sphincter. The secreted bile flows into the duodenum through the common hepatic duct. So-called gallstones (cholelithiasis) that form in the gallbladder or the cystic duct are composed of cholesterol (fatty) substances and bilirubin (lime) substances. In other words, cholesterol and lime in bile accumulate, sediment, and form calculus. Calculus of the cholesterol type forms in the gallbladder. Calculus of the bilirubin type forms not only in the gallbladder, but also in the cystic duct. Passing of this calculus from the cervix of the gallbladder or from the cystic duct into the common hepatic duct results in the condition known as biliary colic (Fig. 99), characterized by fever, pain in the right infracostal region, jaundice, and the appearance of zones (Fig. 100) that are hypersensitive to pressure and often very painful. Cholelithiasis occurs in people who regularly consume large amounts of fat and is characteristic of middle-aged, overweight women.

Since the important thing is to avoid the formation of calculus, one must control the diet by limiting foods high in cholesterol and thus avoid overload on the liver and ensure regular production of bile. In addition, to promote good condition in the liver and the gallbladder, which are intimately related to each other, it is advisable to perform the treatment outlined below regularly.

Shiatsu Therapy

1. When biliary colic develops, the therapist has the patient lie in the right lateral position with both knees bent and brought close to the trunk. Using thumb-on-thumb pressure, he treats the right suprascapular region and the five points in the right interscapular region. Taking point number five in this series as point number one, he treats the three points in the infrascapular region (Figs. 101 through 103). Emphasis should be put on the third, fourth, and fifth points in the interscapular region and the first and second points in the infrascapular region.

2. The therapist moves to the front of the patient's body and, with the digital ball of his right thumb, following the costal border, applies palm pressure to the right inferior costal region (Fig. 104). He directs the force toward the liver and gradually increases pressure. Then he applies vibrational palm pressure.

3. When the pain has subsided, the therapist has the patient lie supine and applies adequate palm or thumb pressure to the area from the diaphragm to the right inferior costal region (Fig. 104).

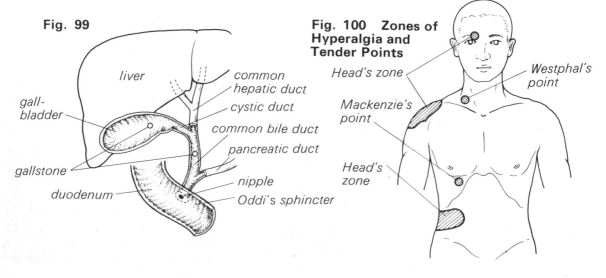

Fig. 99

liver
common hepatic duct
cystic duct
gall- bladder
common bile duct
pancreatic duct
gallstone
nipple
duodenum
Oddi's sphincter

Fig. 100 Zones of Hyperalgia and Tender Points

Head's zone
Westphal's point
Mackenzie's point
Head's zone

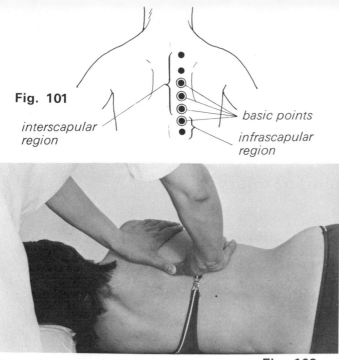

Fig. 101

interscapular region

basic points

infrascapular region

Fig. 103

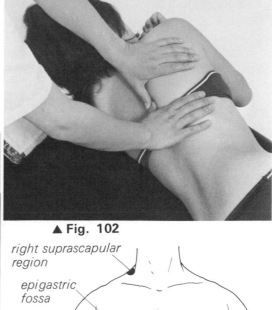

▲ Fig. 102

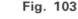

right suprascapular region

epigastric fossa

right inferior costal region

Fig. 104

6. Gastrospasms

Tension in the stomach causes the circular muscles to contract spasmodically, stimulating cramplike pains in the upper abdomen. This condition, which is called gastrospasms, is caused by peptic ulcers, gastritis, or neuralgic stomachache. Other conditions that can bring it about include biliary colic resulting from cholelithiasis, liver ailments, pancreatitis, appendicitis, and arteriosclerosis in the abdominal aorta.

Shiatsu Therapy

1. When the cause of the gastrospasms is irregularity in the stomach itself, the patient lies in the left lateral position; and the therapist repeatedly executes treatment on the left suprascapular region and the five points in the left interscapular region (Fig. 105). Pressure must be applied in concentration on any areas that are especially stiff.

When the cause of the spasms is cholelithiasis or ailments in the liver, the patient lies in the right lateral position; and the therapist treats the right suprascapular region and the five points of the right interscapular region.

2. The patient then assumes the supine position; and the therapist treats the left upper abdominal region and epigastric fossa, if the stomach itself is the cause of the trouble, and the right inferior costal area and epigastric fossa, if the liver or cholelithiasis is the cause (Fig. 106).

3. No matter which of the conditions is the cause, finally, the patient assumes the prone position; and the therapist treats the four infrascapular points (beginning with the fourth interscapular points) on the right and left sides simultaneously. Three seconds of strong pressure are applied to each point (Fig. 107).

Fig. 105

suprascapular region

four points downward from the fourth interscapular point

Fig. 106

epigastric fossa

inferior costal region

Fig. 107

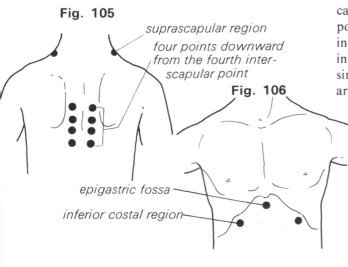

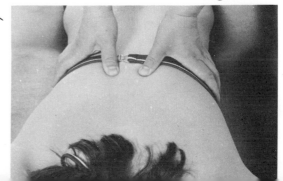

Irregularities in the Locomotor System

1. Whiplash-type Injury (Traumatic Injury to the Cervical Vertebrae)

Passengers in colliding automobiles—especially those in the vehicle that is struck—often suffer violent snapping motions of the head that cause injury in the cervical vertebrae. Following the example of an American orthopedic surgeon who first reported it, most people refer to this condition as whiplash-type injury, though it is more accurately described as traumatic injury to the cervical vertebrae. At first, it assumes the form of a contusion; but later such indeterminate complaints as headaches, insomnia, buzzing in the ears, loss of appetite, pain in the cervical muscles, stiff shoulders, numb arms, and palpitations. The whiplash syndrome of symptoms persists for a long time after the accident that causes them.

At the time of impact caused by the collision, the head is first snapped to the rear (hyperextension of the neck) then it snaps forward in reflex reaction (hyperflexion of the neck) (Figs. 108 and 109). This sudden action gives rise to abnormalities in the muscles, ligaments, blood vessels, nerves, and vertebral disks of the cervical zone. The sudden movement forces the muscles of the neck to overcontract and overextend. This in turn bursts capillaries, setting up inflammation and gradual contracture. As a result of this condition, subluxation of the cervical vertebrae and hernia in the intervertebral disks take place. Then pressure is exerted on the neighboring nerves and blood vessels, and the whiplash syndrome sets in.

Shiatsu Therapy

The first thing that must be done after an automobile collision is to have a physician carefully and thoroughly examine the patient to determine what damage has been done to the neck. Sometimes, depending on the symptoms, immobility is required in cases of whiplash injury; but once inflammation has been taken care of, to prevent persistent aftersymptoms, shiatsu treatment is advisable, for if these symptoms go uncorrected, the patient may fall victim to headaches, insomnia, irritability, and neuroses that aggravate the other conditions. Shiatsu therapy should be employed as soon as it is known that the case involves whiplash injury to prevent aftersymptoms.

1. Having the patient assume the *seiza* kneeling position, the therapist investigates by pressing all of the pressure points in the anterior cervical region, lateral cervical region, medulla-oblongata region, occipital region, suprascapular region, and interscapular region (Figs. 110 through 112) in this order to determine the occurrence of muscular irregularity, swelling, inflammation, and pain. Then he lightly treats the zones discovered to be afflicted in one way or another.

2. Next, having the patient assume first the lateral position, the prone position, and finally the supine position, the therapist performs gen-

Fig. 108 Normal Range of Cervical Region

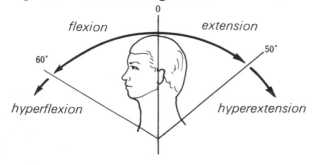

Fig. 109 Hyperflexion and Hyperextension at the Time of Collision

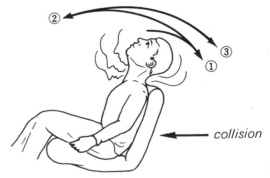

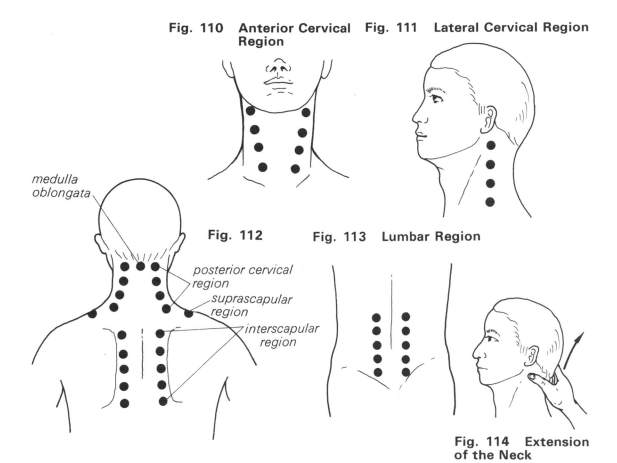

Fig. 110   Anterior Cervical   Fig. 111   Lateral Cervical Region
Region

medulla
oblongata

Fig. 112   **Fig. 113   Lumbar Region**

posterior cervical
region
suprascapular
region
interscapular
region

Fig. 114   Extension
of the Neck

eral shiatsu therapy over the entire body. Treatment must be especially careful and gentle in those locations where there is pain, fever, or swelling. Though, in cases of whiplash injury, attention is usually concentrated on the cervical region, if descriptions of the accident indicate that the lumbar region too is affected, careful treatment should be performed on that zone as well.

3. When this total treatment has limbered the neck, shoulders, and back, the therapist, having the patient once again assume the *seiza* kneeling position, places the thumb of his right hand on the first left lateral cervical point and then the four remaining fingers of that hand on the right first lateral cervical point. Putting his left hand on the patient's frontal region for support, he tilts the head slightly in the posterior direction then extends the whole cervical region upward (Figs. 114 and 115). This extension lasts for five seconds and is repeated three times.

Fig. 115

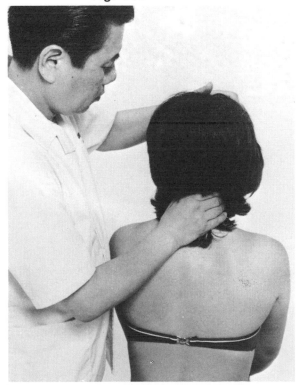

214

2.   Hernia of the Intervertebral Discs

Sudden twists of the trunk cause painful hernias of the intervetebral discs, most readily in the fourth and fifth lumbar vertebrae. The cervical vertebrae are the next most likely to suffer from this affliction. Whether a person is sitting or standing, major body load falls on the lumbar vertebrae. For this reason, the muscles and ligaments attached to these vertebrae are in a state of virtually constant tension. When, as a consequence of this state, they lost resilience and become rigid, pressure is put on the intervertebral discs, which must act as cushions among the vertebrae. The discs too lose resilience. The necleus pulposus immediately behind the center of the intervertebral disc begins to move gradually from the fibrous rings to either the right or the left intervertebral foramen. It is slowly pushed outward. When the discs are in this condition, sudden forward leaning of the trunk causes the nucleus pulposus to slip out of the intervertebral foramen and stimulate pain by coming into contact with the vertebral nerve (Fig. 116).

Though the term *hernia of the intervertebral discs* is used to cover them all, the condition can manifest itself in many different symptoms. Sometimes pain is not severe; sometimes it is so severe that the patient cannot move. It sometimes happens that pain occurs only when the body moves in a certain direction or when the patient walks.

Shiatsu Therapy

1.   First the therapist performs palpation by lightly pressing the area of the spinous processes of the lumbar vertebrae from above with the digital ball of his middle finger. Pain will be caused in the vertebrae in which there is hernia —most commonly in the fourth and fifth lumbar vertebrae (Fig. 117).

He must next investigate to discover whether the hernia is in the right or left transverse process of the spinous process. This is done by carefully pressing with one thumb on top of the other. The place that is in pain is the location of the hernia (Fig. 118).

2.   For the sake of explanation, it is assumed that the hernia occurs in the left side between the fourth and fifth lumbar vertebrae. First the therapist applies thumb-on-thumb pressure immediately below the fourth lumbar vertebra; three seconds per point. The pressure is of an upward kneading kind, and application is repeated from three to five times (Fig. 118). Then he uses downward, thumb-on-thumb pressure on the point immediately above the fifth lumbar vertebra. Pressure lasts for from three to five seconds per point and is repeated from three to five times. Upward kneading and downward pressure are repeated alternately for from three to five times (Fig. 119). This treatment is generally delivered when the patient is in the prone position; but if this is inconvenient, in cases of

Fig. 116

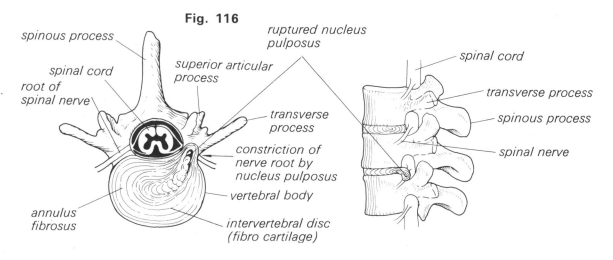

spinous process
spinal cord
root of spinal nerve
annulus fibrosus
superior articular process
ruptured nucleus pulposus
transverse process
constriction of nerve root by nucleus pulposus
vertebral body
intervertebral disc (fibro cartilage)
spinal cord
transverse process
spinous process
spinal nerve

215

Fig. 117 Palpation of the Spinous Process

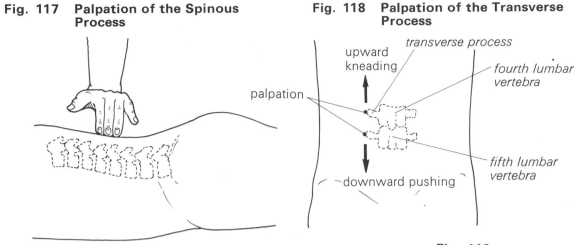

Fig. 118 Palpation of the Transverse Process

transverse process
upward kneading
fourth lumbar vertebra
palpation
fifth lumbar vertebra
downward pushing

Fig. 119

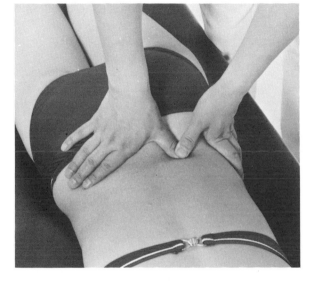

left hernia, the patient may be in the left lateral position and in the right lateral position for cases of right hernia.

3. Having the patient lie supine, the therapist treats the abdominal region, with emphasis on the lower abdomen. Then, putting the digital ball of the left thumb on the left anterior superior iliac spine (right anterior superior iliac spine in the case of the right hernia), he gently and gradually applies vertical pressure then suddenly releases it (Fig. 120). This is repeated from three to five times.

4. When the pain has been relieved enough that the patient can move, the therapist should add to the treatment outlined above therapy on the lumbar region, iliac crest, sacral region, Namikoshi point (Fig. 121), small-intestine

Fig. 120

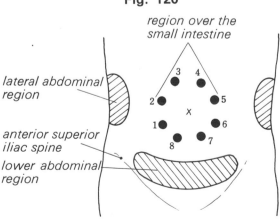

region over the small intestine
lateral abdominal region
anterior superior iliac spine
lower abdominal region

Fig. 121

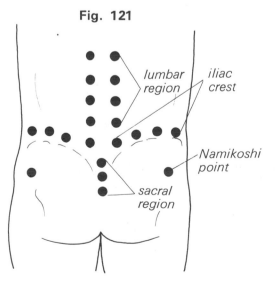

lumbar region
iliac crest
Namikoshi point
sacral region

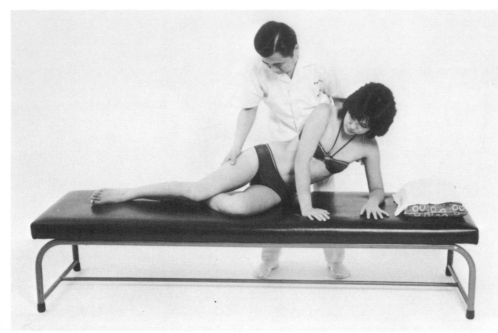

Fig. 122

Fig. 123
▶

Fig. 124

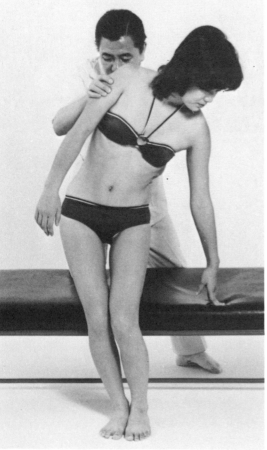

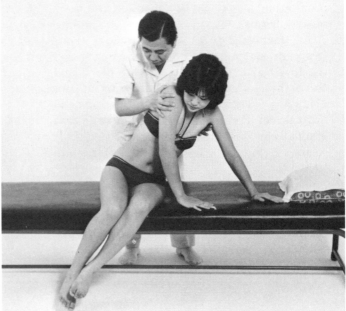

region, lower abdominal region, and lateral abdominal region (Fig. 120). Therapy must be continued for a while even after pain has been completely eliminated.

After the therapeutical session, the therapist must support the patient's trunk and assist her in standing (Figs. 122 through 124). At the start of the session, too, he must help the patient as much as is needed to prevent harmful motion. A treatment table is useful in dealing with patients whose movement is restricted in this way.

3. Mogigraphia (Writer's Cramp)

Mogigraphia, or writer's cramp, is an occupational disability common with people who write by hand a great deal. From the small motions demanded to wield a pen, the muscle groups of

Fig. 125

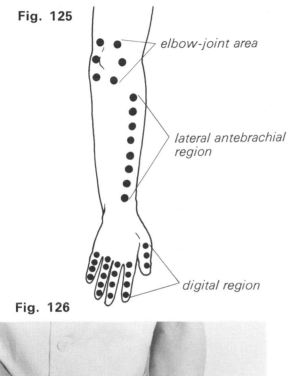

elbow-joint area

lateral antebrachial region

digital region

Fig. 126

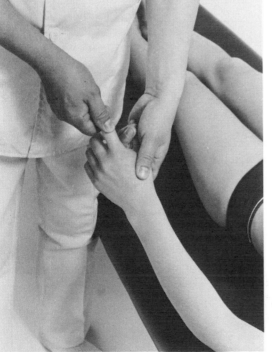

the antebrachial region and the digital tips become fatigued; and, when the person picks up a pen to write, spasms occur. If the person tries to suppress the spasms, trembling starts and makes writing difficult. Frequently worrying about the disabling occupational effect of this condition inspires psychological problems that make matters worse. It is therefore important to calm the patient with the assurance that a full cure is possible as soon as shiatsu relieves fatigue and restores normal contractibility to the muscles.

Shiatsu Therapy

1. With emphasis on the afflicted side, the therapist must carefully treat the entire cervical region, which is usually stiff in patients with mogigraphia.

2. Then he treats the medulla-oblongata region and the suprascapular region.

3. He treats the entire arm on the afflicted side with emphasis on the stiff antebrachial region, the interphlangeal joints, and the dorsal and palmar sides of the hand. He next extends the digits and the arm (Figs. 125 and 126).

4. Great care should be taken to treat the palmar interosseous joints and the dorsal interosseous joints (Figs. 127 and 128).

5. When the area of the elbow joint is stiff, it too must be limbered and softened (Fig. 125).

6. The therapist must perform therapy on the head to calm the patient mentally.

Fig. 127 Treatment for the Volar Interosseous Muscle and Adduction of the Fingers

Fig. 128 Treatment for the Dorsal Interosseous Muscle and Abduction of the Fingers

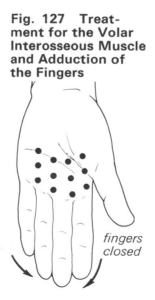

fingers closed

fingers spread

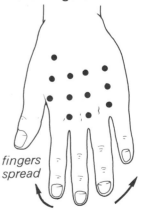

218

4.   Cramps in the Gastrocnemius Muscle

After long hours of standing, mountain climb-
ing, swimming, or running, cramps often occur
in the gastrocnemius muscle. Sometimes, after
a person has gone to sleep, rolling over in bed
will cause such spasms, which are extremely
uncomfortable. Causes may be fatigue, diarrhea,
insufficient water in the blood as a result of
diabetes, venous thrombosis, or varix causing
blood congestion in the crural region.

Shiatsu Therapy

1.   The therapist applies upward-downward,
fluid, and thumb-on-thumb pressure on both
sides of the popliteal fossa (Fig. 129).

2.   Then he uses one-palm pressure and sustained pressure on the gastrocnemius muscle.
Raising the patient's leg at this time increases
the effectiveness of the treatment (Fig. 130).
When the cramps have subsided, he alternates
thumb and palm pressure on the stiff region of
the gastrocnemius muscle.

Once these cramps start, they tend to become
habitual. This should be prevented by taking
care that fatigue does not accumulate and by
self-administered shiatsu at bathing time on the
posterior femoral region, the popliteal fossa, the
sural region, the Achilles' tendon, and the
plantar surface of the foot (Fig. 129).

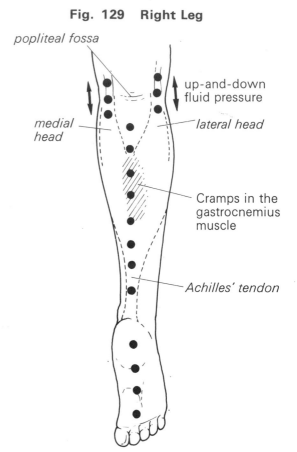

Fig. 129   Right Leg

popliteal fossa

up-and-down fluid pressure

medial head

lateral head

Cramps in the gastrocnemius muscle

Achilles' tendon

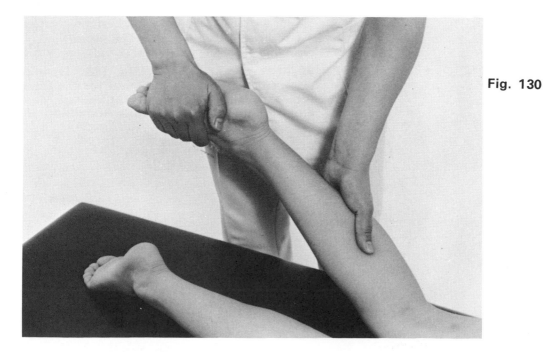

Fig. 130

5.   Stiff Shoulders

Fig. 131

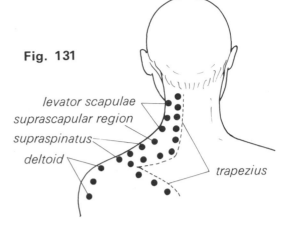

Practically everyone has experienced stiffness in the muscle group running from the cervical region to the shoulders. Though often it results from fatigue in the arms caused by work like lifting and carrying heavy objects, in some instances, the condition is the result of reflexes connected with the internal organs. When something is wrong with the heart or the stomach, a pathological reflex causes stiffness in the left suprascapular region. Irregularities in the liver and gallbladder cause stiffness in the right suprascapular region. This is generally referred to as a cutaneovisceral reflex. Stimulating the surface of the body and thus acting through the muscles

makes it possible to employ the reverse cutaneovisceral reflex to regulate the internal organs. For example, it is well known that pressure on the left suprascapular region will stimulate hunger in a person who suffers from loss of appetite.

Fig. 132

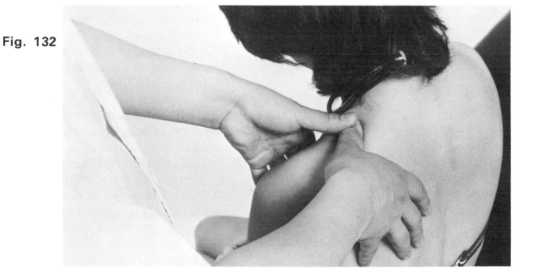

Shiatsu Therapy

When fatigue is the cause, the therapist must thoroughly treat the right and left suprascapular

regions and the trapezius muscle, the levator scapulae muscle, the supraspinatus muscle, and the deltoid muscle (Figs. 131 and 132).

When the cause is reflex from internal-organic disturbance, the therapist must apply concentrated pressure on the suprascapular region of the afflicted side. The pressure must be directed toward the center of the trunk at the height of the seventh thoracic vertebra and must last for five seconds on each point. The effect of this therapy can be greatly improved by performing it as the patient assumes first the *seiza* kneeling position, next the lateral position, and then the prone position (Fig. 133).

Figl 133   Treatment for the Suprascapular Region in the Prone Position

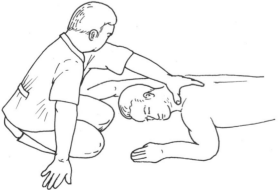

6. Paralysis of the Ulnar Nerve (Claw Hand)

As a consequence of trauma or muscular atrophy in the area controlled by the ulnar nerve, terminal paralysis strikes the flexor muscles of the ulnar side of the antebrachial region, palmar region, and dorsal region causing them to lose mobility and become dysesthetic. When this happens because of paralysis and atrophy in the abductor digiti minimi muscle, the opponens digiti minimi muscle, the flexor digiti minimi brevis muscle, and the palmaris brevis muscle—which con-

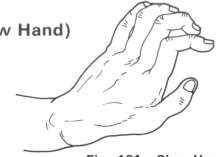

Fig. 134   Claw Hand

stitute the hypothenar—and the dorsal interosseous muscles, the volar interosseous muscles, and the lumbrical muscles, the metacarpal interosseous muscles and the palmar muscles become very thin; and the metacarpal interosseous fossa becomes conspicuous. This condition makes it impossible to bunch the five fingers together or to flex the fingers and hand. When the patient attempts to force his hand to do these things, the metacarpophalangeal joints flex dorsally; and the distal phlanges bend to put the hand in a shape resembling the claw of an eagle (Fig. 134).

Shiatsu Therapy

1. The therapist first treats the six points from the axilla to the medial brachial region and the eight points in the medial antebrachial region on the afflicted side (Figs. 135 and 136).

2. He then treats the lumbrical muscles of the palmar region and the muscle group in the hypothenar (Figs. 135 and 137).

3. Next he treats the whole hand and the dorsal interosseous joints (Fig. 138). By concentrating on treatment of the palmar lumbrical muscles, the therapist strengthens the powers of flexion of the metacarpophalangeal joints and the contractile powers of the dorsal and volmar interosseous muscles and naturally restores ability to open and close the hand.

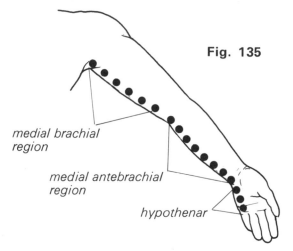

Fig. 135

medial brachial region

medial antebrachial region

hypothenar

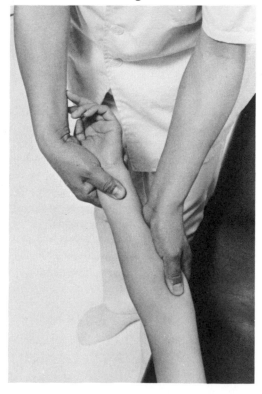

Fig. 136

Fig. 137 Lumbrical and Volar Interosseous Muscles

Fig. 138 Dorsal Interosseous Muscle

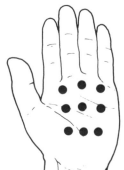

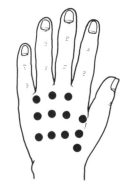

7.　Paralysis of the Median Nerve (Ape Hand)

Damage caused by trauma or muscular atrophy in the median nerve of the arm brings about paralysis and dysesthesia in the region it controls. Paralysis of the median nerve causes atrophy in the abductor pollicis muscles, the flexor pollicis brevis muscle, and the opponens pollicis muscle, which constitute the thenar, thus robbing the thumb of its powers to oppose the other fingers, a power that distinguishes the human hand from the hands of the apes. For this reason, paralysis of the median nerve results in a condition in which the index finger's inability to flex prevents the thumb from reaching the middle finger when the fist is clenched is sometimes referred to as ape hand (Fig. 139).

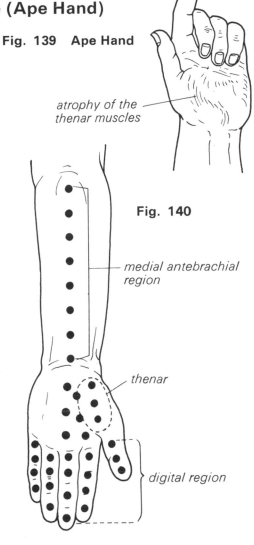

Fig. 139　Ape Hand

atrophy of the thenar muscles

Fig. 140

medial antebrachial region

thenar

digital region

Fig. 141

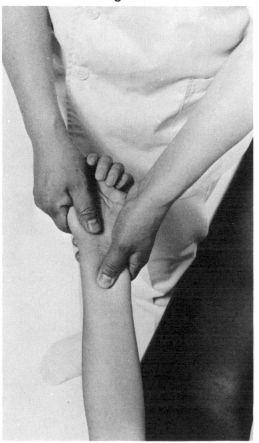

Shiatsu Therapy

1.　First the therapist treats the eight points along the median line of the antebrachial region from the cubital fossa to the wrist joint (Figs. 140 and 141).

2.　Then he thoroughly treats the flexor carpi radialis and palmaris longus muscles running through the center of the palmar region from the wrist joint to the bases of the digits in order to restore their powers of contraction.

3.　Then he shifts pressure from the center of the palm to the thenar to limber the muscles in this region and carefully softens the flexor muscles with special emphasis on the digits and the palmar side.

8. Paralysis of the Radial Nerve (Wristdrop)

Since the radial nerve runs fairly close to the surface of the skin on the lateral side of the humerus at a point about one-third of its way from the bottom, it can easily suffer motor paralysis or dysesthesia as a consequence of trauma, bone fracture, contusions; atrophy; injections; or pressure exerted on it during sleep. When this happens, it is commonly impossible to flex the wrist joint. The condition is not readily apparent when the arm hangs by the body. But, when the patient extends his arm directly to the side with the dorsal side upward, it is impossible for him to straighten his hand, which hangs limply at roughly right angles with the antebrachial part of the arm (Fig. 142). Furthermore, the patient is unable to bring his hands together in the prayerful attitude, since the afflicted hand will drop downward from the tips of the digits.

Fig. 142   Wristdrop

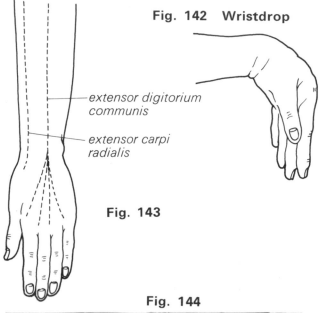

extensor digitorium communis

extensor carpi radialis

Fig. 143

Fig. 144

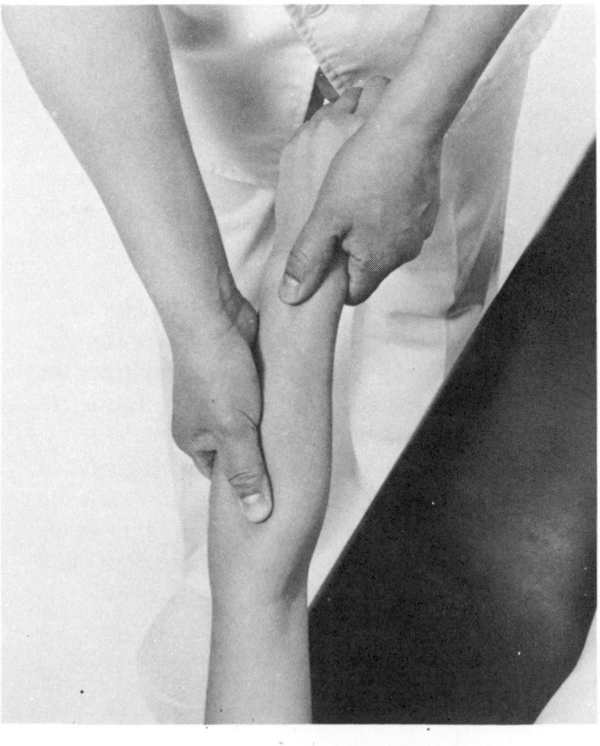

Shiatsu Therapy

1.   The therapist treats the lateral brachial region of the afflicted arm in the area through which the radial nerve passes and the area slightly lower with sustained pressure.

2.   After thoroughly limbering the first point on the lateral antebrachial part, he treats the eight points leading from there to the wrist joint in order to return the extensor digitorum communis muscle to normal functioning (Figs. 143 and 144).

3.   He treats the extensor carpi radialis muscle of the wrist joint thoroughly.

4.   Then he has the patient raise the arm straight from the shoulder joint above the head and flex the wrist joint dorsally (Fig. 145). This must be repeated slowly several times.

5.   Finally, holding the digits of the patient's hand in both of his own hands, the therapist extends and vibrates them for ten seconds. This is repeated several times.

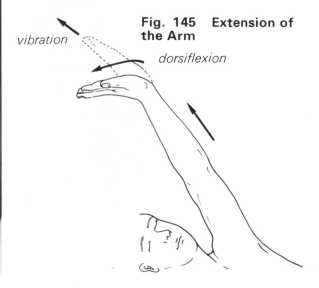

vibration

Fig. 145   Extension of the Arm

dorsiflexion

9. Prosopoplegia (Facial Paralysis)

When trauma, cold, thrombosis, or rheumatism cause paralysis in the motor nerves controlling facial expression, the action of the mimic muscles become erratic; and the face is distorted. But, since this condition, called prosopoplegia or facial paralysis, affects the motor, and not the sensory, nerves, it is accompanied by no pain.

Symptoms vary with the location of the paralysis. For instance, if the orbicularis oris muscle at the mouth is affected, the afflicted side will lose its powers of contraction with the result that it is pulled in the direction of the sound side, leaving the mouth half open. A patient with this condition is unable to whistle because he can not pucker his mouth to the same extent on both sides. He will drool in his sleep. When the orbicularis oculis muscle is affected, the patient is unable to close the afflicted eye entirely, even while sleeping.

Shiatsu Therapy

1. The therapist must execute one full course of facial shiatsu treatment.

2. Next, using either his thumbs or his index, middle, and ring fingers, he applies either ordinary or sustained pressure on the paralyzed area. To restore the contractile powers of the muscles, when the mouth—for example—is being treated, he must move pressure points at small intervals and apply suction pressure in a pulling direction from the sound side toward the afflicted one (Figs. 146 and 147).

Fig. 146 Suction Pressure with Three Fingers

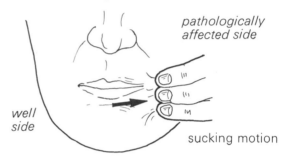

Fig. 147

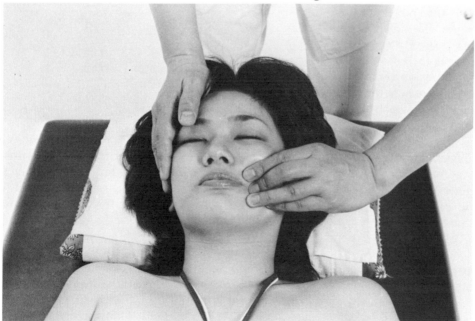

10. Scapulohumeral Periarthritis (Frozen Shoulders)

This condition occurs in the shoulder—a universal joint with the greatest motion latitude of any joint in the body—especially in people who are about fifty years of age. The shoulder joint is surrounded with a synovial bursa and encased in muscles and ligaments (Figs. 148 and 149). People suffering from this affliction suddenly experience sharp pain when performing abduction, external rotation, or extension of the shoulder to the rear in putting on a jacket or gripping the suspended support straps on trains. The pain causes unnaturalness in all of the body motions. If this condition is allowed to persist for a long time, the deltoid muscle atrophies, the shoulders lose their natural roundness, and motor disability results.

Many causes and symptoms are lumped together under the term scapulohumeral periarthritis. Deformation of the joint, muscular degeneration, adiposis, adhesions, inflammation of the synovial bursa, and calcipexy are some of them.

Shiatsu Therapy

1. Beginning with treatment of the suprascapular region, the therapist presses the supraspinatus muscle in the direction of the outer side of the deltoid muscle (Figs. 150 and 151).

2. Then he presses the infraspinatus muscle from the interscapular region toward the outside. In the same way, he limbers the teres minor muscle, the teres major muscle, the latissimus dorsi muscle, and the axilla by applying pressure to them.

3. Next he presses at small intervals on the outer part of the round area of the deltoid muscle (middle fibers). Then, concentrating on the places where pain occurs, he treats the anterior region (anterior fibers) and posterior (posterior fibers) of the same muscle (Figs. 152 and 153).

4. Since outer rotation of the shoulder joint is one of the motions that is most restricted by scapulohumeral periarthritis, the therapist has the patient raise his arm, bend his elbow, and put his hand on his occipital or posterior cervical regions.

Fig. 148   View of the Top of the Left Shoulder Joint

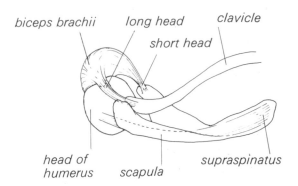

Fig. 149   Posterior Surface of the Left Shoulder Joint

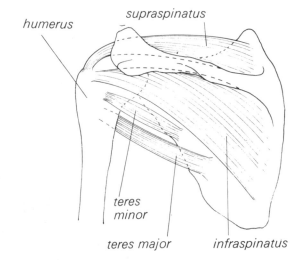

Even when the condition has not advanced to scapulohumeral periarthritis, sluggishness in the region of the deltoid muscles and cracking sounds as the shoulder is rotated outward indicate the initiation of contracture in the muscles and tendons. To prevent the situation from getting worse, it is advisable to limber this area by means of self-administered shiatsu and to perform such exercises as turning, rotating, and lifting the shoulder to the rear regularly. Shiatsu in the region of the left and right suprascapular regions and the deltoid muscle helps prevent not only scapulohumeral periarthritis, but ordinary stiff shoulders as well.

Fig. 150

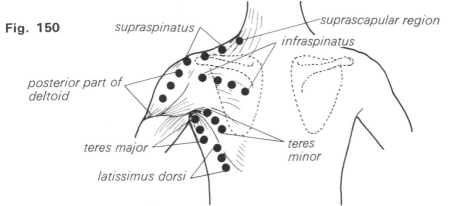

supraspinatus

suprascapular region

infraspinatus

posterior part of deltoid

teres major

latissimus dorsi

teres minor

Fig. 151

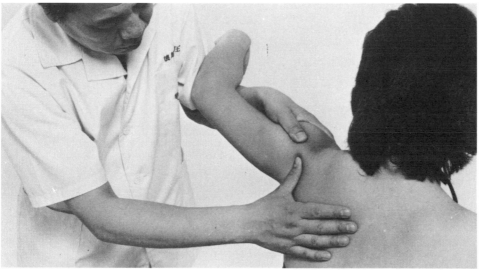

Fig. 152

Fig. 153 ▶

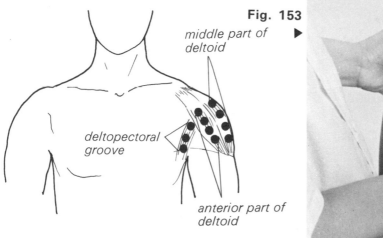

middle part of deltoid

deltopectoral groove

anterior part of deltoid

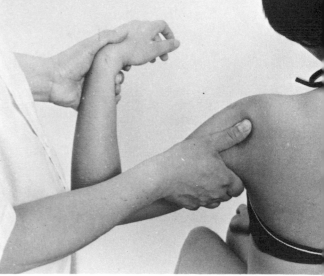

Disorders in the Metabolic, Endocrine, Urinary, and Reproductive Systems

1. Diabetes Mellitus

Insulin secreted by the islets of Langerhans in the pancreas makes it possible for the body to use blood sugar as a source of energy. Blood sugar left over after this process has been carried out is stored in the liver as glycogen. When secretion of insulin is impaired for one reason or another, blood sugar fails to be assimilated and builds up in the blood to be excreted together with urine. This condition is called diabetes, which is one of the so-called adult diseases. Though said to be related to heredity, diabetes often afflicts people who eat too much and too well, who are overweight, and who are deficient in the insulin needed to assimilate excess sugar. Some of the symptoms of the sickness are sugar in the urine, which has a fruity odor; loss of energy; sharp

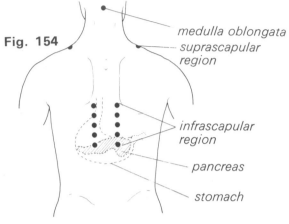

Fig. 154

medulla oblongata
suprascapular region
infrascapular region
pancreas
stomach

reduction in weight, though the person has formerly been obese; thirst, unusually frequent urination; weakening eyesight; loss of skin luster; and itching.

Shiatsu Therapy

1. Having the patient assume the prone position, the therapist thoroughly treats the medulla-oblongata region, the suprascapular regions (especially the five points in the right and left interscapular region, and the infrascapular region (Figs. 154 through 156).

2. Having the patient assume the supine position, the therapist treats the lower abdominal region. Since the pancreas is located directly behind the stomach, it is especially important to soften the stomach thoroughly to prevent its applying pressure on the pancreas.

Fig. 155

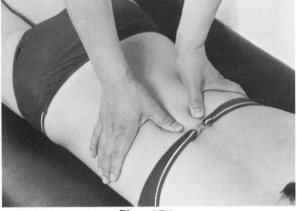

Fig. 156

Fig. 157

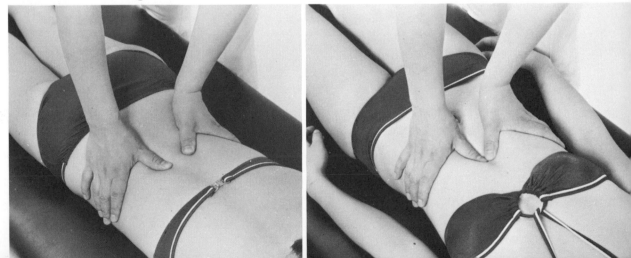

2. Gout

Though gout was virtually unknown in Japan earlier, after World War II, when the Japanese diet began to improve, it began to appear, particularly in middle-aged men who tend to be overweight and who eat a great deal of meat and drink alcoholic beverages in considerable quantity.

Under ordinary circumstances, the protein known as purine bodies is easily dissolved and passed out of the body as uric acid through the kidneys. But when these bodies are too plentiful, uric-acid metabolism fails; and uric acid remaining in the body creates deposits of uric-acid salts around joints sometimes to the extent that the bone is destroyed and intense pain results. This condition often occurs in the first metatarsophalangeal joint of the big toe (Figs. 158 and 159). It causes fever and intense pain often throughout the night.

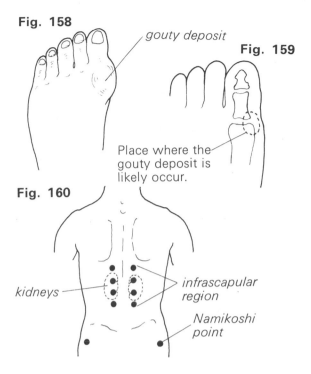

Fig. 158

gouty deposit

Fig. 159

Place where the gouty deposit is likely occur.

Fig. 160

kidneys

infrascapular region

Namikoshi point

Shiatsu Therapy

1. Having the patient lie in the prone position, the therapist treats both sides of the spinal column from the interscapular to the lumbar region, with special attention to points three, four, five, and six in the infrascapular region (Fig. 160) since these are at the position of the kidneys. He first uses palm pressure and then thumb pressure (Fig. 162).

2. He treats right and left Namikoshi points simultaneously.

3. Taking care not to touch the swollen, painful part, he treats the bottom of the foot, especially the five points in the arch (Figs. 162 and 163).

4. Having the patient lie in the prone position, the therapist carefully treats the lateral crural region and the entire abdominal region.

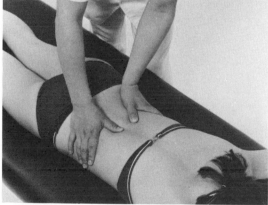

Fig. 161

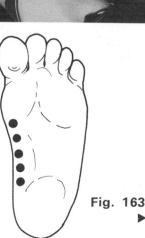

Fig. 162   Plantar Region

Fig. 163

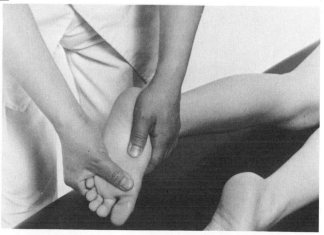

3. Kidney Disorders

The kidneys are located on either sides of the vertebral column between the eleventh thoracic and the third lumbar vertebrae. The right kidney tends to be somewhat lower than the left one. Shaped like beans, ten centimeters long and five centimeters wide, they are capped with the suprarenal bodies. Their major function is to filter wastes from the blood and discharge them with urine without losing useful elements and maintaining balance in the blood.

Arteriosclerosis, liver disorders, or high blood pressure can increase the load on the kidneys, cause metabolic irregularities, and result in such sicknesses as nephritis, cirrhosis of the kidney, nephrolithiasis (calculus in the urinary tract), and nephrosis. Excesses of water and salts in the body caused by these conditions generally manifest themselves as albuminuria and edema. In the early stages, swelling occurs, especially in the upper eyelid. The swelling results from the accumulation of body fluids among the thin subcutaneous tissues and connective-tissue membranes. As the sickness progresses, dents made in the crest of the tibia at the anterior crural region by manual pressure fail to fill out quickly when pressure is released. Called pitting, this condition is used in the diagnosis of kidney disorders.

Fig. 164 Infrascapular-lumbar region

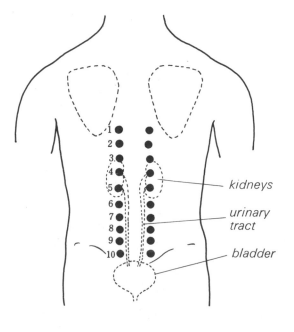

Shiatsu Therapy

1. Having the patient assume first the left lateral, then the right lateral, and finally the prone position, the therapist varies his pressure as he treats the ten points from the infrascapular to the lumbar region. Since the points near the kidneys—3, 4, 5, and 6 (Fig. 164)—are hard, gentle pressure should be applied slowly to them (Fig. 165).

2. Then interlocking the fingers of both hand, he presses simultaneously both kidney regions, using the bases and palms of both hands. Applications last five seconds (Fig. 166). After repeating this, he applies vibrational pressure.

3. Having the patient remain in the prone position, the therapist lightly treats the legs. Bending the patient's knees, he treats the right and left arches simultaneously (Fig. 167). While doing this, he causes the knees to flex still further until the heels approach the gluteal region. This must be repeated several times.

4. Having the patient assume the supine position, he carefully treats the anterior surfaces of the legs. Finally, he carries out full treatment of the abdominal region.

Fig. 165

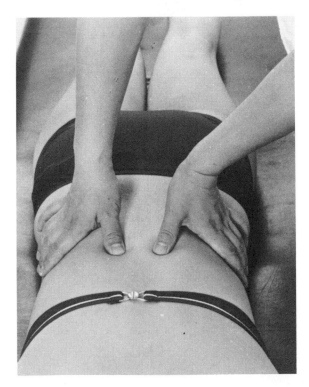

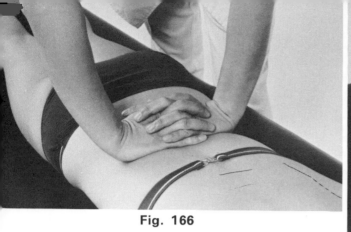

Fig. 166

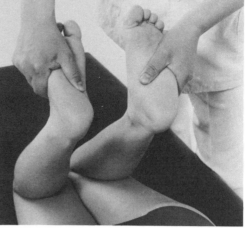

Fig. 167

4. Hypertrophy of the Prostate Gland

Part of the male reproductive system, the prostate gland, which is about the size of a chestnut, is located to the rear and below the bladder at the base of the urethra facing the rectum (Fig. 168). The fluid secreted by the prostate gland, along with the secretion of the testes, the epidermis, the spermatic duct, and the seminal cyst, is one of the elements of seminal fluid. For causes related to the endocrine system, one sign of aging in men of more than sixty years is a pathological hypertrophy of the prostate gland, which obstructs urination, though the sufferer is frequently awakened several times during the night with the urge to urinate. The most important factor in caring for this condition is early prevention by means of a regular system of shiatsu therapy to keep the body in good condition.

Shiatsu Therapy

1. First the therapist presses the point in the medulla-oblongata region (Fig. 169) five or six times; pressure lasts for from six to seven seconds per application. This stimulates the medulla oblongata and helps maintain endocrine balance.

2. Having the patient assume the prone position, the therapist treats the right and left lumbar regions and the Namikoshi points (Fig. 169) simultaneously. Strong pressure is used on the Namikoshi points. Then he treats the three sacral points; pressure is applied to each five or six times.

3. Having the patient assume the supine position, he treats the lower abdominal region with palm pressure lasting five seconds per point. Then he applies either thumb pressure or pressure with the index, middle, and ring fingers on the position at the pubic bone located directly above the bladder.

4. Finally, with both palms or with the index, middle, and ring fingers of both hands he applies vibrational pressure for ten seconds and repeats the application five times

Fig. 168   Male Sexual Organs

Fig. 169

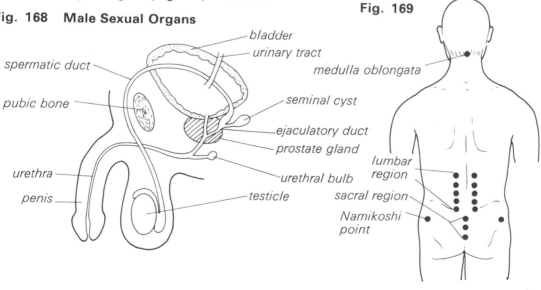

spermatic duct

pubic bone

urethra

penis

bladder
urinary tract
medulla oblongata
seminal cyst
ejaculatory duct
prostate gland
urethral bulb
testicle
lumbar region
sacral region
Namikoshi point

5. Impotence

The impotent male is unable to have an erection or to complete sexual intercourse. Though there are many reasons for the condition, psychological causes often play the most important role: psychological tension, stress, insecurity in relation to sexual matters, memories of failure in initial sexual intercourse, premature ejaculation, and complexes about the body. Consequently, ensuring emotional balance and ridding the patient of stress are the first steps in treatment. In addition, a nourishing diet and adequate sleep are vital.

Shiatsu Therapy

1. Beginning with the anterior cervical region, the therapist treats the entire cervical region.

2. Having the patient lie in the prone position, the therapist carefully treats the medulla-oblongata region; the suprascapular region; and the dorsal, lumbar, and sacral regions (Figs. 170 and 171). Then he treats the Namikoshi points.

3. Having the patient assume the supine position, the therapist limbers the entire abdominal region. He takes special care to apply repeated sustained pressure with the thumbs and palms on the area of the pubic bone (Figs. 172 and 173). Accompanying this with palm pressure on the inguinal region increases the effectiveness of treatment.

Fig. 170

Fig. 172

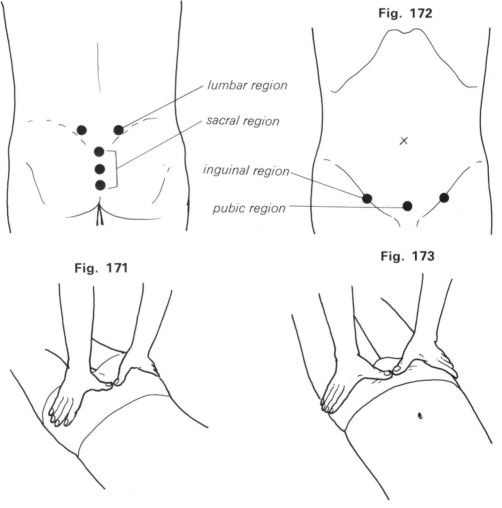

lumbar region

sacral region

inguinal region

pubic region

Fig. 171

Fig. 173

6. Agenesia

Inability to have children is the fault of the male in roughly fifty percent of all cases and of the female in roughly fifty. In the instance of the male, congenitally underdeveloped testes or malformation or other irregularity in the sperm may be the cause. Inflammation of the testes as a consequence of epidemic parotitis can cause male sterility if it strikes after puberty. In females, causes of barrenness include malfunction of the ovaries, underdevelopment of the uterus, obstruction of the uterocervical canal, and abnormal ovum. Inflammation of the ovaries can occur in females who are afflicted with epidemic parotitis after the initiation of puberty.

Still, many married couples are unable to have children, though both partners are apparently free of physical defect. In these cases, psychological elements are usually the cause. Stress or tension upsets the autonomic nervous and endocrine systems. Shiatsu examinations in instances of this kind reveal stiffness in the cervical and lumbar regions in both males and females. The degrees of stiffness of the right and left gluteal regions are sometimes different, because displacement of the sacroiliac joint twists the pelvis. This condition causes reduced functioning of splanchnic nerves of the pelvis in the parasympathetic nervous system—from the pelvis to the reproductive organs, the descending colon, the rectum, and the bladder—and consequent imperfect functioning of the reproductive system. When this is the case, the lower abdomen is generally stiff and chilled.

Shiatsu Therapy

1. Treatment begins with the cervical region. In this order, the therapist thoroughly limbers the anterior cervical region, lateral cervical region, medulla-oblongata region, and posterior cervical region.

2. Having the patient assume the prone position, he treats the dorsal region, with special attention to both sides of the vertebral column in the lumbar region, the iliac crest, the sacral re-

Fig. 174

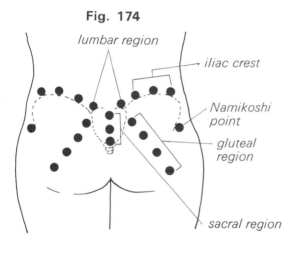

lumbar region

iliac crest

Namikoshi point

gluteal region

sacral region

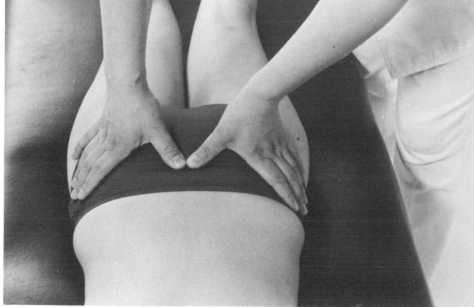

Fig. 175

Fig. 176

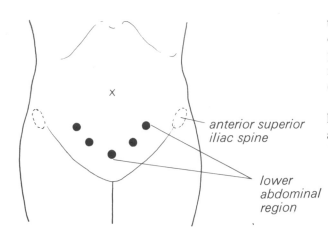

anterior superior
iliac spine

lower
abdominal
region

gion, the gluteal region, and the Namikoshi point (Figs. 174 and 175).

3. Having the patient assume the supine position, the therapist treats the right and left anterior superior iliac spine alternately with vertical pressure applied with the thenar in order to restore the sacroiliac joint to normal condition (Figs. 176 and 177).

4. Next he thoroughly relieves stiffness in the lower abdomen by means of sustained pressure applied with either the thumbs or the palms (Fig. 178).

Fig. 177   **Fig. 178**

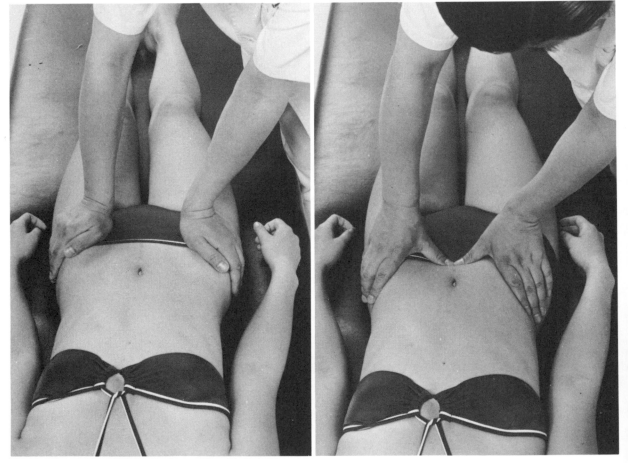

7. Chilling

Even when the weather is not especially cold, women sometimes complain of localized chilling in the cervical region, the scapular and dorsal regions, the lumbar region, the joints of the legs and arms, extremities of the legs and arms, and the lower abdominal region. The causes are irregularities in the autonomic nervous system dulling the action of the vasomotor nerves, which in turn create obstructions in the circulation and abnormalities in endocrine secretions. Loss of appetite, indigestion, anemia, chilling at night, and menstrual pains frequently accompany chilling.

Shiatsu Therapy

It is important to improve blood circulation and put the body in better condition by treating all parts likely to be subject to such chilling, with special attention to the parts where the patient complains of chilling (Figs. 179 and 180): anterior cervical region; medulla-oblongata region; posterior cervical region; suprascapular region; interscapular region; lumbar region; sacral region; gluteal region; Namikoshi point; legs (especially the lateral crural region, posterior crural region, dorsal region, plantar region, and digits of the feet); arms (especially the lateral antebrachial region, dorsal region, digits, and palmar region of the hands); abdomen (especially the lower abdomen—Fig. 180).

Fig. 179   Shiatsu Points on the Back at a Place Where Chilling is Likely to Occur

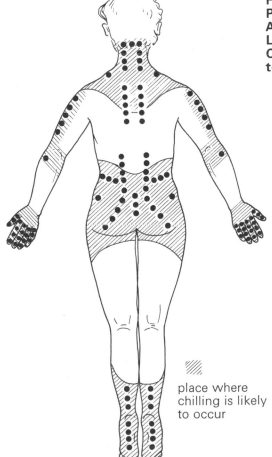

place where chilling is likely to occur

Fig. 180   Shiatsu Points on the Abdomen at a Location Where Chilling is Likely to Occur

Fig. 181

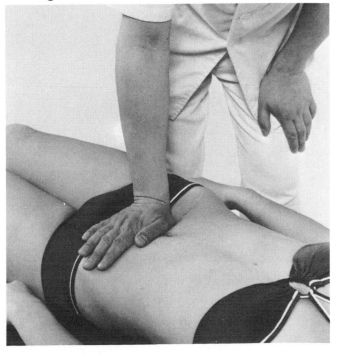

8. Morning Sickness

Morning sickness, manifesting itself in loss of appetite, nausea, increased salivation, vomiting, and alterations in dietary preferences, is a pregnancy condition usually occurring in the second or third month. As the name indicates, it frequently strikes early in the morning before the expectant mother has had anything to eat.

It is thought that chorionic tissues dispose of metabolic products at the time of the formation of the placenta. These products enter the blood stream, alter the constituent elements of the blood, and thus bring about the condition called morning sickness, which usually terminates in the fourth month of pregnancy, when the placenta has been fully formed. Severe or persistent cases of morning sickness (known as hyperemesis gravidarum) tend to occur in people with weak stomachs and in neurotic people.

Shiatsu Therapy

In treating pregnant women, the therapist must perform therapy lightly. Obviously the prone position is out of the question; and all therapy must be performed in the seated position, the right or left lateral positions, or the supine position. It should never be performed when the patient's stomach is empty. After meals, when the stomach is settled, is the best time.

1. Having the patient sit straight, the therapist lightly treats the anterior, lateral, and posterior cervical regions and the medulla oblongata.

2. Having the patient assume the left lateral position, he carefully limbers the stiff suprascapular and interscapular regions. Then he slowly and carefully softens the especially hard points in the series of points from the fourth intersacpular to the third infrascapular (Figs. 182 and 183). He then lightly presses all points from there to the tenth infrascapular points (lumber region). Having the patient assume the right lateral position, the therapist performs the same treatment on the right side.

3. Having the patient lie in the supine position, he lightly and slowly applies palm pressure to the entire abdominal area, with special emphasis on the epigastric fossa.

When appetite develops during pregnancy, the woman should take small amounts of easily digested food at any time she likes. Since vomiting reduces body fluids, she should drink more cool, refreshing drinks, tea or milk, than usual to stimulate urination, which removes poisons from the body. She should always remain calm and remember that, no matter how unpleasant the condition is, morning sickness is only temporary.

Fig. 182   From the Fourth Interscapular Point to the Third Infrascapular Point

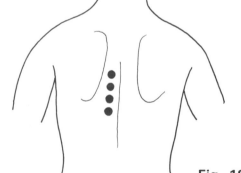

Fig. 183

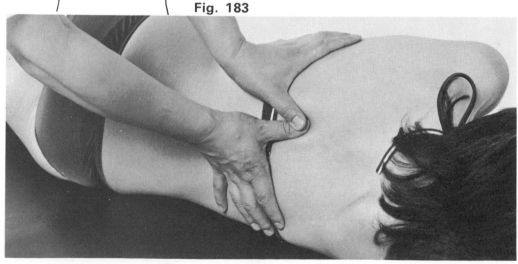

9. Climacteric Upsets

Though there are individual differences among people, almost all women experience cessation of monthly menstruation at the time of menopause, or the climacteric. When this happens, the ovaries function at a reduced rate; and the balance of the endocrine system is upset with the result that the autonomic nervous system is disturbed, causing stress, increased blood pressure, headaches, palpitations, and other symptoms. The troubles are more severe with thin, nervous women and with women who tend to suffer from chills. Since they are strongly influenced by psychological elements, the more the woman worries about them, the longer these symptoms are likely to persist. Consequently, it is of the utmost importance for the woman to remain calm and to reassure herself that the difficulties will pass with time.

Shiatsu Therapy

1. Having the patient assume the left lateral position, the therapist treats the left cervical regions; the anterior cervical region, the lateral cervical region, the medulla-oblongata region, and the posterior cervical region. He then has the patient assume the right lateral position and repeats the same therapy on the right side. In this treatment, emphasis is placed on the anterior cervical and medulla-oblongata regions.

2. Having the patient assume the prone position, the therapist applies thorough treatment to the occipital region, the suprascapular region, the lumbar region, and the Namikoshi point (Fig. 184). Next he lightly treats the legs.

3. Having the patient assume the supine position, the therapist lightly treats the anterior surfaces of the legs, the arms, the head, the facial region, and the entire abdomen. Special attention should be paid to treating the lower abdomen and the epigastric fossa and to palm pressure on the eyes (Figs. 185 and 186).

Fig. 185

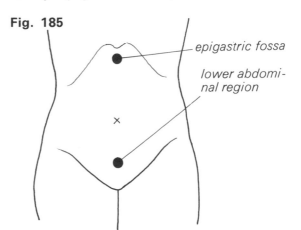

epigastric fossa

lower abdominal region

Fig. 184

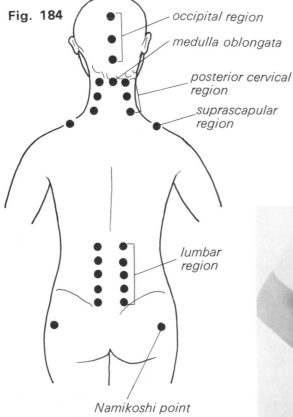

occipital region

medulla oblongata

posterior cervical region

suprascapular region

lumbar region

Namikoshi point

Fig. 186

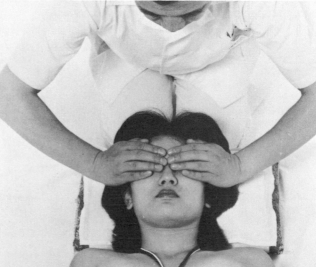

Fig. 187

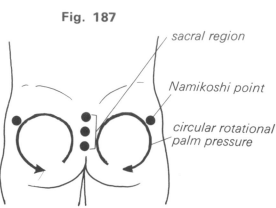

sacral region

Namikoshi point

circular rotational palm pressure

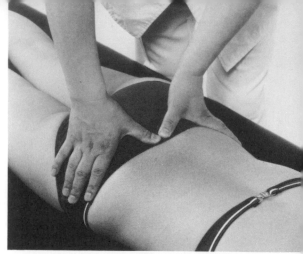

Fig. 188

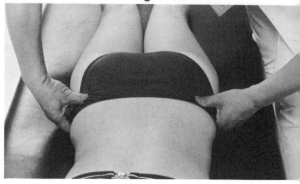

Fig. 189

10. Irregular Menstruation and Menstrual Pains

Ordinarily women menstruate once in a period averaging twenty-eight days, but sometimes the cycle is disturbed. Some women go for long periods without menstruating; some young women fail to initiate menstruation at the normal age. Most often menstrual irregularities arise from hormone imbalance caused by psychological tension or shock, from constitutional weakness or excess fatigue, or from pathologically induced bodily weakness. Ordinary menstruation causes most women to experience menstrual pains in the lower abdomen, pain in the lumbar region, headaches, and nausea. In severe cases, the afflicted woman must rest from work and domestic duties. In these instances, the uterus is insufficiently developed; or its excess retroflexion or anteflexion causes pain when it contracts strongly during menstruation.

Shiatsu Therapy

1. Having the patient lie in the prone position, the therapist applies repeated simultaneous treatment to the right and left sides of the medulla-oblongata region, the lumbar region, the sacral region, and the Namikoshi points. Pressure applications last five seconds per point (Figs. 187 through 189).

2. Several applications of circular palm pressure (outwardly directed) are alternately performed on the right and left gluteal regions (Fig. 187).

3. Having the patient assume the supine position, the therapist alternately treats the right and left anterior superior iliac spines. Then, with vertically directed pressure applied with the thenar, he thoroughly limbers the lower abdominal region (Figs. 190 and 191).

Fig. 190 Lower Adbominal Region

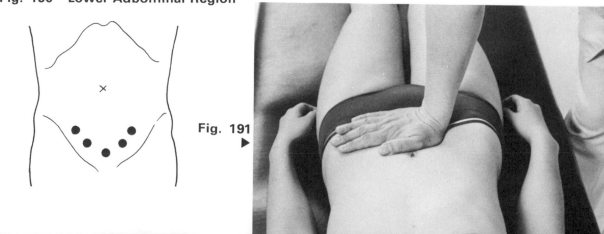

Fig. 191
▶

Disorders in the Sensory Organs

1. Blepharoptosis (Drooping of the Upper Eyelids)

Blepharoptosis is a condition in which the upper eyelids droop heavily (Fig. 192), forcing the afflicted person to wrinkle the forehead, raise the eyebrows, and thrust the chin forward in order to see upward. In severe cases, the patient must manually lift his eyelids to see. The condition results from paralysis in the levator palpebrae superioris muscles on one or both sides of the face and resultant closing of the palpebral fissure. Though often the trouble is congenital, it can be caused by trauma or abnormalities in the oculo-motor nerves or underdevelopment of the levator palpebrae superioris muscles. In adults, chronic eyestrain or lid edema causes the condition.

Shiatsu Therapy

1. Having her lie in the prone position, the therapist moves behind the patient's head. He applies sustained pressure with the index, middle, and ring fingers of his hands to the patient's closed levator palpebrae superioris muscles.

2. Then with the same three fingers or with the thumb he presses on five points, at short intervals, on the levator palpebrae superioris muscles. The pressure is applied with a slight pull in the direction of the frontal region (Figs. 193 and 194). He then uses vibrational pressure. In both instances, he takes care not to press directly on the eyeballs.

Fig. 192

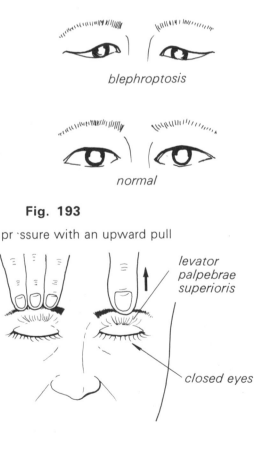

blephroptosis

normal

Fig. 193

pr·ssure with an upward pull

levator palpebrae superioris

closed eyes

Fig. 194

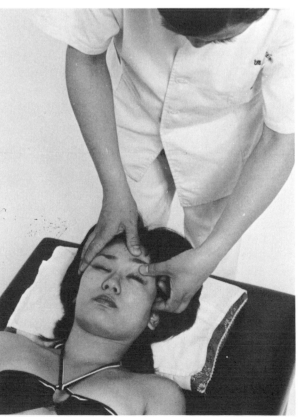

2. Sinusitis

The condition known as sinusitis is an accumulation of pus in the paranasal sinuses—pneumatic space continuous with the nasal cavity, such as the maxillary sinus, frontal sinus above the glabella, ethmoidal sinus between the nose and eyes, and sphenoidal sinus on the eye median line (Fig. 195)—caused by inflammation from catarrh or other infectious ailments. The stuffy, heavy feeling that this condition brings on can cause insomnia and greatly reduces powers of concentration, recall, and thought. Sometimes the condition is acute (for instance, as when caused by catarrh); but in others it is the chronic result of allergy.

Fig. 195   Position of the Paranasal Sinus

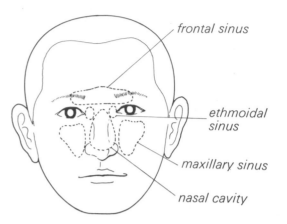

frontal sinus

ethmoidal sinus

maxillary sinus

nasal cavity

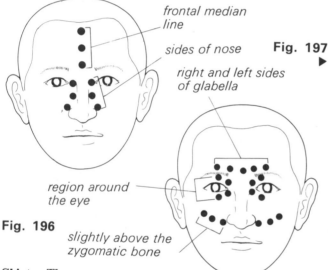

frontal median line

sides of nose

Fig. 197 ▶

right and left sides of glabella

region around the eye

Fig. 196

slightly above the zygomatic bone

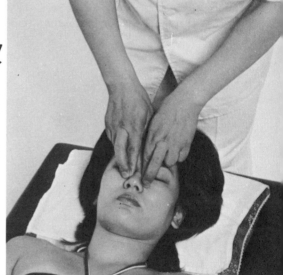

Fig. 198

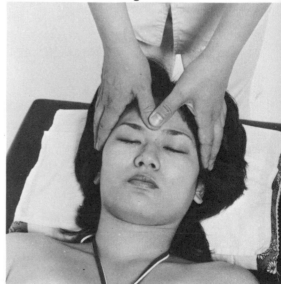

Shiatsu Therapy

1.   Having the patient assume the left lateral position, the therapist thoroughly treats the medulla-oblongata and posterior cervical regions to stimulate the sympathetic nerves and thus to cure inflammation by causing contraction in the blood vessels of the nasal mucous membrane. When this happens, nasal breathing becomes free and normal again.

2.   Having the patient assume the supine position, the therapist concentrates on the median line of the head and applies pressure to the frontal median line, the periphery of the orbicular zone, both sides of the nose, and the area slightly above the zygomatic border (Figs. 196 through 198).

Fig. 199

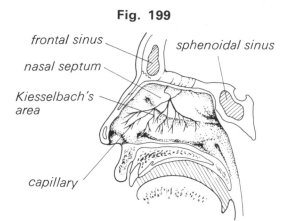

frontal sinus
nasal septum
Kiesselbach's area
sphenoidal sinus
capillary

3. Epistaxis (Nosebleed)

In children, the numerous small blood vessels in the nasal mucous membrane are so sensitive and fragile that a simple blow on the nose can cause them to erupt and thus bring about the condition called epistaxis or nosebleed. Sometimes eating chocolate or drinking beverages high in caffein content stimulates these blood vessels to expand and burst so that the nose bleeds. The location called the Kiesselbach's area in front of the nasal septum (Fig. 199) is most likely to be the source of nasal hemorrhage. In adults who suffer from arteriosclerosis, high blood pressure, or other ailments that make blood vessels fragile, epistaxis can occur. In addition, it is often a compensation occurrence in menstruation or cerebral hemorrhage.

Shiatsu Therapy
Having the patient assume the seated position, the therapist treats the region of the medulla oblongata (Figs. 200 and 201). Then, holding a clean handkerchief or towel against the patient's nose with his left hand, the therapist presses with his right thumb against the medulla-oblongata region. Pressure is thrusting and upward kneading and is directed toward the nasal septum (Figs. 202 and 203). It lasts for from five to seven seconds and is repeated. Such pressure stimulates the center of vasoconstriction in the medulla oblongata to cause blood vessels to contract and thus effectively stops nasal hemorrhage.

Fig. 200   Effects of the Treatment on the Medulla Oblongata

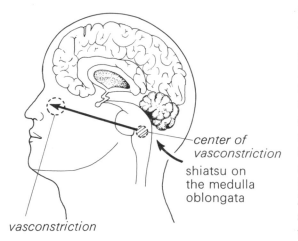

center of vasconstriction
shiatsu on the medulla oblongata
vasconstriction

Fig. 201

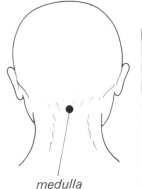

medulla oblongata

Fig. 202   **Fig. 203**

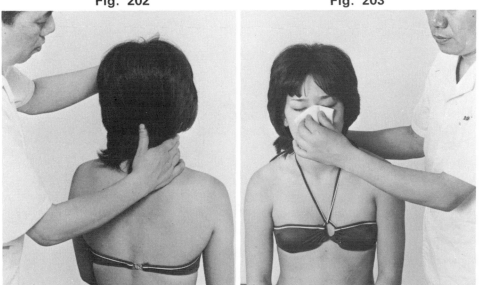

4. Motion Sickness

Vibration, up-down motion, and variation of the speeds of automobiles, ships, and aircraft cause people—most often young girls—to suffer motion sickness, which manifests itself in dizziness, nausea and possible vomiting, cold sweat, and facial pallor. The movement of the vehicle causes variations in the pressure of the lymph spaces in the labyrinth, or inner ear. This in turn stimulates the sensory epithelium, upsets the balance of the autonomic nervous system, and results in the symptoms outlined above. The condition is common in people with weak stomachs, gastroptosis, insomnia, and nervous hypersensitivity.

Since motion sickness is related to auditory, visual, and olfactory senses, people who are prone to it should read or listen to music while riding and try to keep their eyes off the outdoor scenery as it flashes past. The dry air inside a tightly enclosed vehicle stimulates the nasal mucous membrane. Since this is not good, people who are victims to this condition should slowly sip steamy, hot drinks or hold moist, hot towels against their noses when riding. Because anxiety about falling victim to it frequently brings on the condition itself, it is of the utmost importance to remain calm.

Shiatsu Therapy

1. Having the patient sit upright and placing his left palm on her forehead as support, the therapist slowly and calmly treats the lateral cervical region, the medulla-oblongata region, and the posterior cervical region with his left hand (Figs. 204 and 205).

2. Having the patient assume the prone position, the therapist treats the right and left suprascapular and interscapular regions. He must pay special attention to the fourth and fifth interscapular points (Fig. 204).

3. Finally, having the patient assume the supine position, coordinating his action with her breathing, he applies pressure to the epigastric fossa. If conditions make it impossible for the patient to assume the supine position, she should sit upright; and the therapist should treat the epigastric fossa while standing behind her or to her right side with his right palm.

Fig. 204

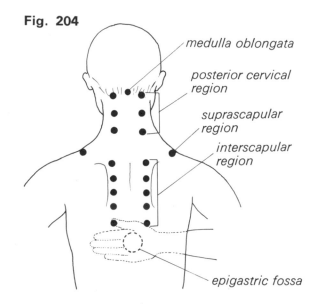

medulla oblongata

posterior cervical region

suprascapular region

interscapular region

epigastric fossa

Fig. 205

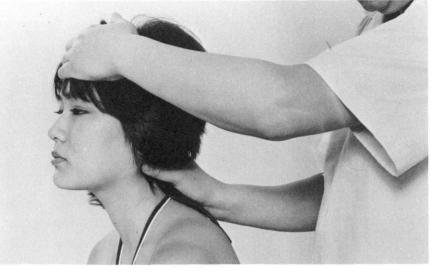

5. Tinnitus (Buzzing in the Ears)

Buzzing in the ears may be unilateral or bilateral. Unilateral buzzing is a pathological condition in the external and middle ear. Bilateral buzzing is a condition of the inner ear and is related to other bodily illnesses. Buzzing in low tones is a condition of the middle and outer ear, whereas buzzing in high tones is a condition of the inner ear. Among the several causes are high blood pressure, low blood pressure, arteriosclerosis, climacteric troubles, rheumatism, insomnia, Ménière's disease, the Ménière's syndrome, anemia, foreign objects in the external ear, cerumen, and so on. As a result of some of these causes, the blood vessels in the vicinity of the ear contract; and the pulsation of these vessels is heard in the ears. But, in many instances, buzzing is the result of indeterminate complaints. This is often true in instances of unilateral buzzing, when the sound persists for long times.

Shiatsu Therapy

1. Having the patient assume the seated position, the therapist uses his thumbs to press the three points on the anterior, superior, and posterior auricular muscles (Fig. 206).

2. Placing one thumb over the tragus to close the auditory canal (ear hole), he presses the three points around the mastoid process (Fig. 206) for five seconds each. While doing this, he alternately presses and releases the thumb over the auditory canal to open and close the ear (Fig. 207). When this treatment is self-applied, the patient should open and close the auditory canal with the index finger and press the points around the mastoid process with the thumb (Fig. 208).

3. Next the entire ear should be pressed for five seconds lightly with the palm. When the five seconds have passed, the palm must be quickly released. In instances of bilateral buzzing, the palm treatment is applied to the right and left ears simultaneously.

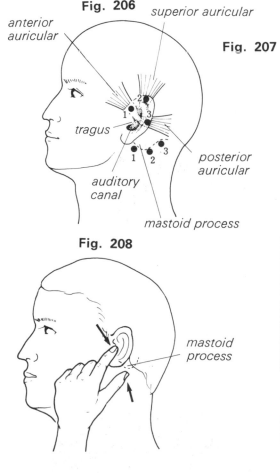

Fig. 206

anterior auricular

superior auricular

tragus

auditory canal

posterior auricular

mastoid process

Fig. 207

Fig. 208

mastoid process

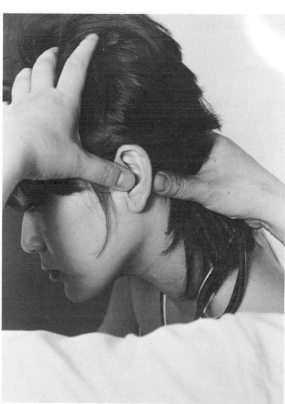

Respiratory Ailments

1. Bronchial Asthma

An asthmatic attack takes the form of sudden stuffiness in the throat, heaviness in the chest, gasping, panting, and persistent coughing. Spasms in the smooth muscles of the bronchial-tube walls bring about a condition called bronchostenosis, which results in expiratory dyspnea. The attacks tend to occur frequently late at night and in the early morning and in the autumn. Asthma is closely related to allergies to foods and things breathed through the mouth and nose. Asthmatic people are hypersensitive in the bronchial passage and esophagus. Though many things to which they are allergic can be listed—dust indoors, pollen, buckwheat chaff, molds, animal hair, crabs, shrimp, buckwheat, eggs, mackeral, spinach, *matsutake* mushrooms, and so on—there is much individual variation.

Shiatsu Therapy
When the patient suffers an attack, she should be instructed to sit up straight for treatment. Characteristic of asthmatic attacks is difficulty in expiration. Expiratory dyspnea caused by the attack makes it impossible for the patient to breathe except in a seated position. This condition is called orthopnea.

1. The therapist begins by applying thumb pressure to the four points in the left anterior cervical region and then the four in the right anterior cervical region (Figs. 209 and 210). This is done slowly and is repeated several times to calm the spasms in the bronchial tubes.

2. Then treatment is applied six times each to the medulla-oblongata region and the right and left posterior cervical regions (Figs. 211). The thumbs are used on the medulla-oblongata region; the thumb and four fingers are used to treat the right and left posterior cervical regions simultaneously.

3. Then the therapist treats the right and left suprascapular region and the five points in the interscapular region (Figs. 212 and 213).

4. Standing behind the patient, the therapist wraps his hands around her upper body so that index, middle, and ring fingers of both hands come into contact on the patient's sternal body.

Fig. 209 Four Points in the Anterior Cervical Region

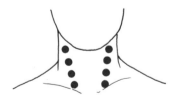

Fig. 210

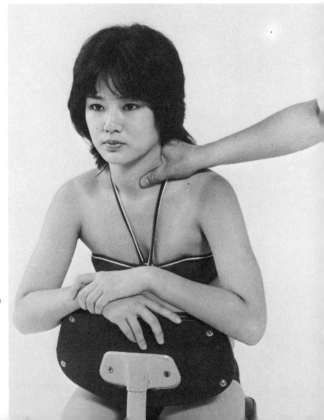

Fig. 211

medulla oblongata

posterior cervical region

Fig. 212

suprascapular region

interscapular region

Fig. 213

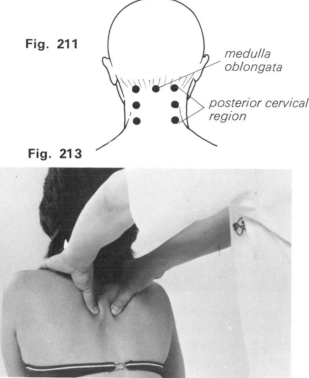

Fig. 214

sternal region
intercostal region

epigastric fossa

Fig. 215

deltopectoral groove

Fig. 216

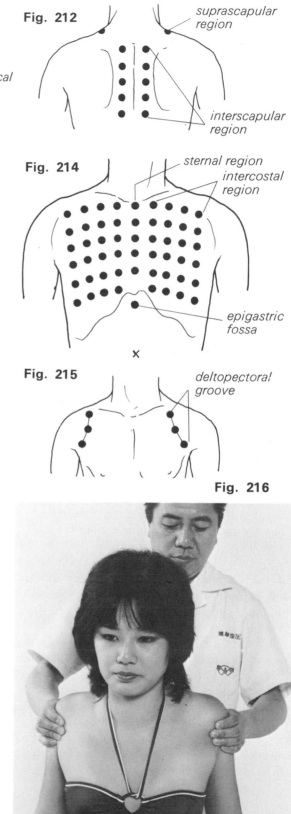

He then treats the five points on the sternal body from top to bottom and repeats the treatment three times (Fig. 214). There are four vertical rows of six points in the intercostal thoracic region on each side of the sternal body.

5. The therapist continues by using the index, middle, and ring fingers of both hands to treat these eight rows, working from top to bottom, simultaneously. This must be performed carefully and repeated from three to five times.

6. Next he uses the same three fingers of both hands to treat the three points on each deltopectoral groove. Treatment is applied with a rearward pull and is repeated six times (Figs. 215 and 216).

7. Finally, once again standing behind the patient, the therapist uses either overlapping palms or index, middle, and ring fingers of both hands held to touch each other and presses the epigastric fossa (Fig. 214) rhythmically six times, three seconds per application. When he presses, he has the patient exhale. When he releases pressure, he has her inhale. This regulates breathing. The numbers of repetitions and degrees of pressure for each of these operations must be gauged to the conditions and the individual patient.

2. Hiccups

Fig. 217

Hiccups are a condition that disturbs practically everyone at one time or another. In medical terms, they are a spastic repetitive respiratory movement called singulation. Nervous tension or the sudden drinking of something hot or eating of something strongly stimulative can bring it about. At the time of swallowing, the phrenic nerve is stimulated, causing spasmodic contraction of the diaphragm and sudden opening of the glottis with an accompanying sound considered characteristic of hiccups.

Hiccups in children can usually be cured by a drink of water and a gentle patting or stroking of the back. In old people, however, the condition can become chronic. To prevent this, it is important to conduct regular shiatsu therapy on the anterior cervical region, dorsal region, and diaphragm.

Shiatsu Therapy

1. Having the patient assume the supine position, the therapist treats the four points in the left anterior cervical region (Fig. 217) and gives special attention to the third point (Fig. 219), through which the phrenic nerve passes. (This treatment is effective in stopping sudden spasms.) Then he treats the four points in the right anterior cervical region in the same way.

2. Having the patient assume the prone position, the therapist treats the three points in the right and left interscapular regions (Fig. 218).

3. Pressing his palms against both of the patient's lateral abdominal regions at the height of the diaphragm, he executes rapid upward and downward applications of suction pressure on the right and left sides at the same time (Fig. 218).

4. Once again having the patient assume the supine position, the therapist gives thorough palm-pressure treatment to the abdomen and executes rapid, upward squeezing motions on both sides of the patient's body at the same time (Fig. 219). This is repeated five times.

All of the treatments outlined above must be adjusted to the individual case and repeated as often as needed. Palm pressure over the eyeballs

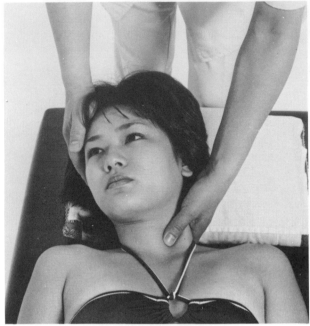

too may be added. Holding the breath while pinching the nose and thrusting the tongue out of the mouth for an extended period are simple methods sometimes used to cure hiccups.

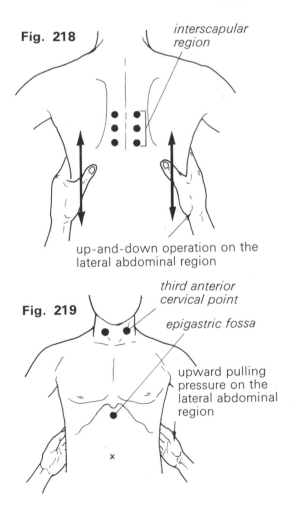

Fig. 218

interscapular region

up-and-down operation on the lateral abdominal region

Fig. 219

third anterior cervical point

epigastric fossa

upward pulling pressure on the lateral abdominal region

Children's Diseases

1. Congenital Myogenic Torticollis

The normal position of the embryo within the uterus is with the neck contracted and the head tucked inward to the chest and oriented downward toward the uterine orifice (Fig. 220 A). In cases of agrippa (breech presentation) or in instances when the embryo face is turned as shown in Fig. 220 B (face presentation), at birth, pressure is put on either the right or the left sternocleidomastoid muscle with a resultant rupture of capillaries in the muscular fibers. The hematoma in the muscle in which this degenerative change occurs grows harder and becomes a neoplasm. As the muscle grows, contracture in the form of a cicatricial cord occurs. The sternocleidomastoid muscle of the afflicted side is shortened, causing the head to lean in the direction of that side and setting up torsion in the sound side (Fig. 221). This condition is called congenital myogenic torticollis and deserves special care since it is often accompanied by congenital dislocation of the hip joint.

Shiatsu Therapy

1. The patient assumes the prone position. With the index and middle fingers, the therapist gently palpates the sternocleidomastoid muscle

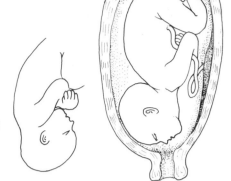

A. Normal attitude   B. Abnormal attitude
(face presentation)·

Fig. 220   Positions of the Fetus

from the head of the sternum to the mastoid process to ascertain the presence or absence of neoplasms or rigidity.

2. When such hardness is located, with the same two fingers, he performs upward-downward, fluid pressure applications at small intervals at the stiff zone (Fig. 222). Depending on the shape of the neoplasm, it may be necessary to grip the afflicted zone between the thumb and index finger to relieve contracture. Without applying too much pressure, the therapist carefully treats the entire anterior cervical region.

3. When the stiffness has been thoroughly relieved, he holds the temporal regions in both hands and gradually turns the head from the afflicted to the sound side (Fig. 223) and then slowly returns it to the original position.

Though contracture of the sternocleidomastoid muscle is easiest to relieve in newborn infants, at this stage, the greatest skill and maturity are demanded of the therapist. Treatment must be extremely cautious and must be left entirely to trustworthy specialists. When such specialists are unavailable, the procedure outlined above should be carried out once a day. But individual therapy sessions must not last too long. If shiatsu treatment is performed regularly and carefully, the ability of the muscle to contract will increase as the child grows older.

Fig. 221

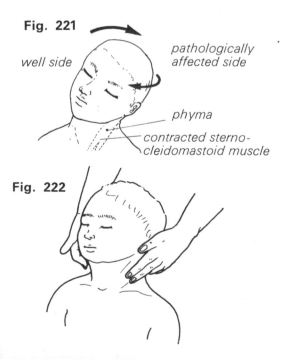

well side

pathologically affected side

phyma

contracted sterno-cleidomastoid muscle

Fig. 222

Alternating rotation from the pathologically affected side to the well side

Fig. 223

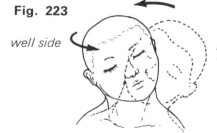

well side

pathologically affected side

2.   Congenital Dislocation of the Hip Joint

Abnormal positioning of the legs of the embryo in the uterus causes slacking in the hip joint. This or imperfect formation of the acetabulum results in dislocation of the head of the femur (Fig. 224). At birth, the head of the femur moves beyond the labrum acetabulare; or, if the condition does not reach this stage, subluxation takes place. Even when everything appears normal at birth, if these conditions are present, sooner or later dislocation or at least slippage is likely to occur.

Congenital dislocation of the hip joint is more common in female infants and more frequent on one side only. Cases of dislocation of both hip joints are rare. Since the head of the femur slips upward and outward, in infants afflicted with this condition, the affected leg is short and marked with conspicuous wrinkles of the skin (Fig. 225). For this reason, at diaper-changing time abduction of the afflicted thigh is limited. Medical examinations to determine dislocation of the hip joint employ the Trendelenburg's symptom. When the infant can walk and stands on only the leg in which the dislocation has taken place, the gluteus maximus and gluteus medius muscles contract incompletely, causing sagging in the buttock on the afflicted side. To compensate and maintain balance, the child leans the upper body in the direction of the afflicted side.

Fig. 225   Posterior Surface of the Buttocks

head of the femur dislocated from acetabulum

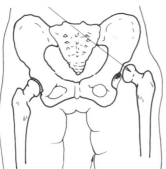

Wrinkles are numerous because of constriction of the leg.

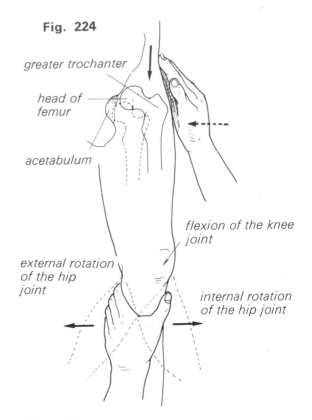

Fig. 224

greater trochanter

head of femur

acetabulum

flexion of the knee joint

external rotation of the hip joint

internal rotation of the hip joint

Shiatsu Therapy

The explanation given below is for dislocation of the left hip joint. Treatment is the same for the right hip joint.

1. Having the patient assume the prone position, the therapist thoroughly limbers the muscle group around the hip joint, especially the gluteus maximus, the gluteus medius, and the tensor fasciae latae muscles (Fig. 226).

2. Having the patient assume the supine position, the therapist carefully palpates the greater trochanter to investigate the position of the dislocation. When the position has been determined, he puts the center of his right palm on the location of the greater trochanter. Then, after having the patient bend her knee and put her hip joint in a forty-five degree angle, he places his left palm on the lower part of the posterior crural area for support. With suction-pressure action of his right palm, he pulls the greater trochanter toward the acetabulum. When the head of the femur has approached the ace-

Fig. 227

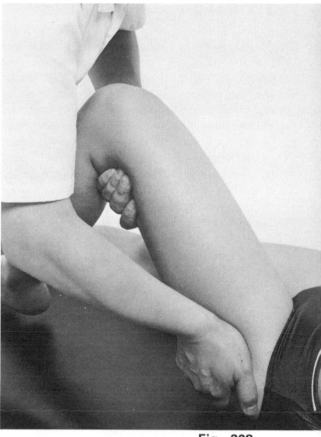

Fig. 226 Posterior and Lateral Surfaces of the Buttocks

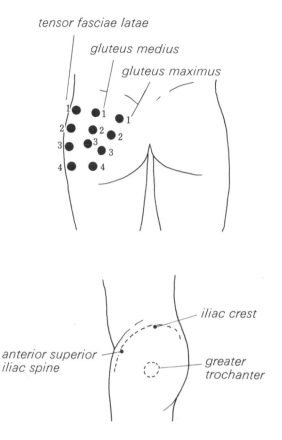

tensor fasciae latae

gluteus medius

gluteus maximus

iliac crest

anterior superior iliac spine

greater trochanter

Fig. 228

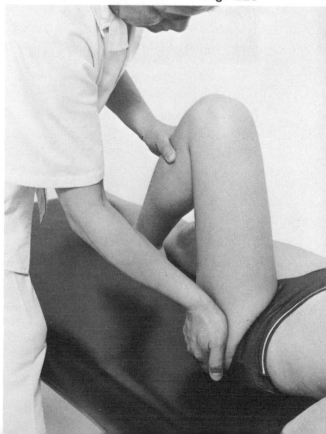

tabulum, he stabilizes it by applying pressure from the lateral direction (Figs. 224 and 227).

3. Leaving his right palm on the location of the head of the femur, he brings his right hand to the anterior crural region. Holding the head of the femur in place with his right palm, with his left hand he pushes the bent knee outward to cause the head of the femur to rotate inward (Fig. 228). This should return the head of the femur to the acetabulum. If pushing the crural area medially and then laterally and rotating the head of the femur laterally and medially produce no abnormal sounds, the joint has been restored to normal. But, since the muscles in the vicinity of the hip joint are still weak, there is great likelihood of recurrent luxation or slippage. For this reason, it is important to continue treatment to strengthen the muscles and stimulate development of the bone.

3. Genu Varum (Bowlegs)

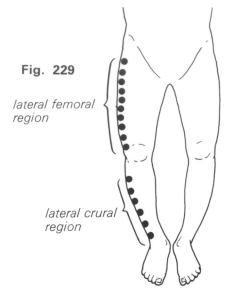

Fig. 229

lateral femoral region

lateral crural region

Though this condition is apparent in the supine position, it is all the more evident when the patient stands. The legs bow outward; that is, the femoral regions turn outward, and the crural regions turn inward. The heels come together, but the tips of the toes do not. Because of the outward curvature, this condition is referred to as O-shape bowed legs. Such bowing is physiologically normal until the third year after birth.

Bowlegs occurs easily in children who are forced to stand prematurely and in those whose bones have not developed properly. In addition, rickets and muscular contraction can be causes.

Fig. 230

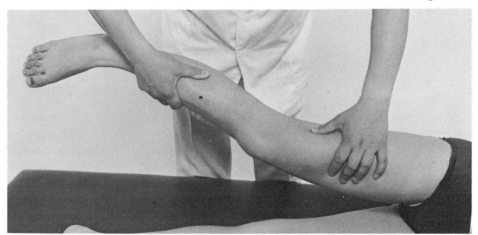

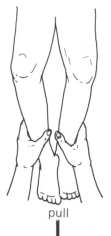

Fig. 231 Extension of the Legs

pull

Shiatsu Therapy

1. Having the patient lie in the supine position, the therapist presses the ten points in the lateral femoral region and the six in the lateral crural region on both legs. This is done as if to bring one leg close against the other (Fig. 229).

2. Having the patient assume the lateral position and supporting the crural region with one hand, the therapist raises the leg. With the free hand, he applies pressure—directed straight down—on the lateral femoral region (Fig. 230). This operation is performed slowly several times.

3. Once again having the patient assume the supine position, the therapist grips each ankle in one hand and simultaneously pulls them (Fig. 231).

4. Genu Valgum (Knock-knees)

The reverse of bowlegs, this malformation involves inward bending of the femoral and outward bending of the crural regions. The tips of the toes come close together, but the heels do not. The condition is sometimes referred to as X-shape knock-knees. Some of the possible causes include rickets, abnormal bone development, muscular contraction, congenital malformation, and poliomyelitis. In cases in which the last is the cause, however, often only one knee is bent.

Shiatsu Therapy

1. Having the patient lie in the supine position, the therapist treats the area of the knee joint.

2. Bending the patient's legs outward at the knees, he applies laterally directed pressure on the ten points in the medial femoral region (Fig. 232).

3. Returning the patient's knees to their original position, the therapist rotates the entire leg inward and treats the six points in the posterior crural region (Fig. 233).

4. Having the patient assume the lateral position, the therapist puts one hand on the medial femoral region for support and with the other hand presses the six points in the posterior crural region.

5. With the leg still raised, the therapist pulls the medial femoral zone upward with one hand while pushing the lateral crural region downward with the other (Fig. 234). This is done gradually and slowly and is repeated several times. This treatment is performed on both legs.

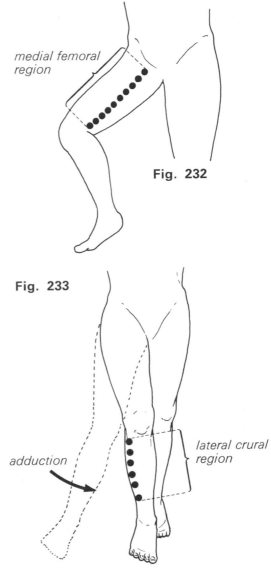

medial femoral region

Fig. 232

Fig. 233

adduction

lateral crural region

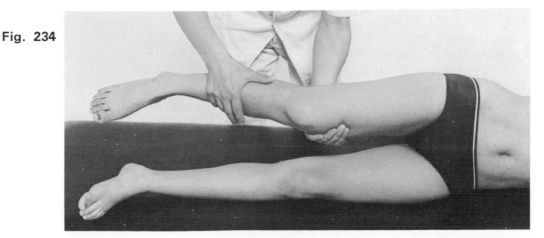

Fig. 234

Fig. 235

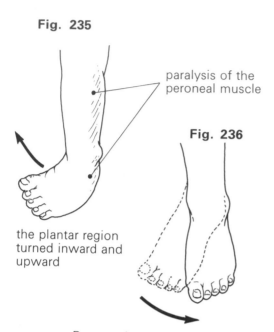

paralysis of the
peroneal muscle

Fig. 236

the plantar region
turned inward and
upward

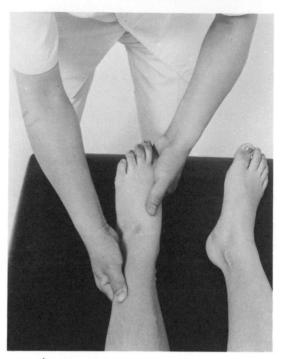

▲ Fig. 237

Pressure is applied to turn the foot outward.

5. Talipes (Clubfoot)

Congenital talipes ranks with congenital torti-collis and congenital dislocation of the hip joint as one of the three most frequent infant deformities. In afflicted children, at birth, the foot is bent inward, the whole foot is twisted, or the plantar region is turned upward medially. The condition generally results from paralysis of the peroneal muscle group (Fig. 235). Poliomyelitis or traumatic injury can account for acquired talipes.

Shiatsu Therapy

1. Thorough pressure treatment is used on the peroneal muscle group, including the peroneus longus, peroneus brevis, and peroneus tertius muscles. During this treatment, with his free hand, the therapist turns the foot as far outward as possible (Figs. 236 and 237).

2. He then presses the lateral part of the ankle, the lateral malleolus, and the dorsal region of the foot (Fig. 238). Special attention must be paid to the dorsal area on the side of the little toe.

3. Bending the patient's knee and putting the plantar region flat on the floor, the therapist

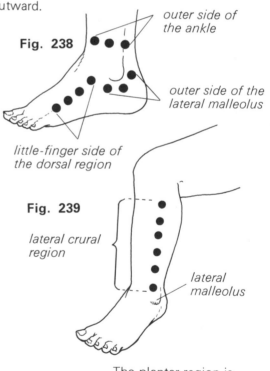

Fig. 238

outer side of
the ankle

outer side of the
lateral malleolus

little-finger side of
the dorsal region

Fig. 239

lateral crural
region

lateral
malleolus

The plantar region is
pressed against the floor.

presses the six points on the lateral crural region (Fig. 239). Since this condition is extremely difficult to correct, therapy must be applied patiently over a long period.

6. Idiopathic Scoliosis

Pathological curvature of the spine to the right or left, the condition referred to as idiopathic scoliosis, occurs often in girls in puberty, between the ages of ten and fifteen, when muscular and skeletal development is most vigorous. When considerably advanced, the condition results in the shape seen in Fig. 240. Even when the person attempts to stand straight—as in the military position of attention—there is a gap between the arm and the side; and the spinal column is not equidistantly related to both scapulae. The malformation is more apparent when the person first stands straight then bends the trunk forward (Fig. 241). The definite causes are unknown, but parents must be especially watchful for spinal curvature in their teenage children. Scoliosis is easier to deal with if caught in an early stage. Prevention can take the form of a good, balanced diet and adequate, correct exercise to keep the muscles nourished and limber.

Shiatsu Therapy

1. Since stiffness of the muscles in the cervical region causes the head to lean to one side, the therapist begins by having the patient either sit straight or assume the formal kneeling (*seiza*) position and by pressing the anterior cervical region, lateral cervical region, medulla-oblongata region, and occipital region (Fig. 240). He should limber the muscles in these regions thoroughly.

2. He must then give adequate attention to thumb-pressure treatment applied alternately to the left and right suprascapular and interscapular regions.

3. The therapist grips each of the patient's wrist joints with his hands and raises the arms straight above the patient's head. He then causes the patient to bend the trunk rearward. This must be done lightly at first, as a warm-up. Then, when the patient has relaxed this part of the body, the same treatment should be repeated several times to extend the trunk thoroughly.

Fig. 240

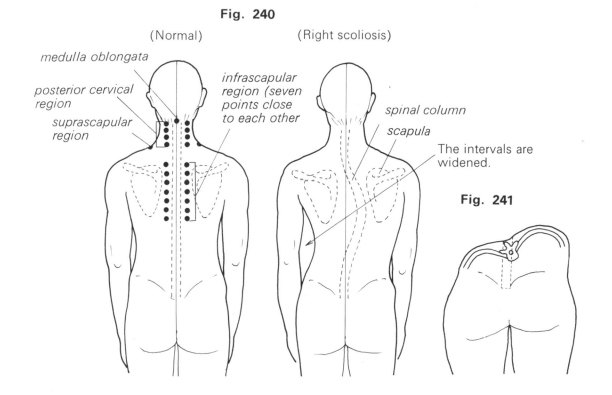

(Normal)   (Right scoliosis)

medulla oblongata

posterior cervical region

suprascapular region

infrascapular region (seven points close to each other

spinal column

scapula

The intervals are widened.

Fig. 241

Fig. 242 Flexion and Extension of the Trunk

Fig. 243 Lateral Flexion of the Trunk

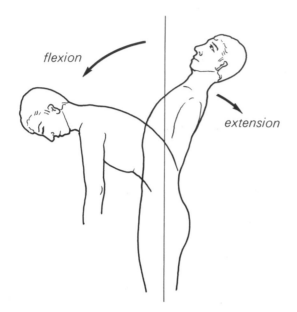

flexion

extension

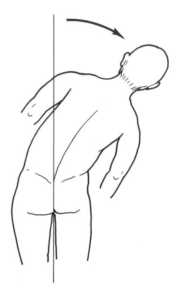

Performed daily for from five to ten minutes, this exercise prevents the occurrence of spinal curvature and stops mild cases from getting worse. Self-administered shiatsu and daily exercise to extend, bend, and rotate the trunk will not only prevent spinal curvature, but also stimulate growth and invigorate the functioning of the internal organs.

Fig. 244 Rotation of the Trunk

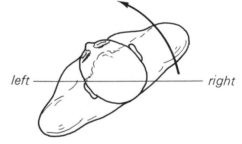

left —————————————— *right*

Index